Basta!

Basta!

A Doctor's Story of Giving Back

DARIUS R. MAGGI, M.D.

BASTA!

A Doctor's Story of Giving Back

ISBN 978-1-61961-469-7 *Paperback*

978-1-61961-470-3 *Ebook*

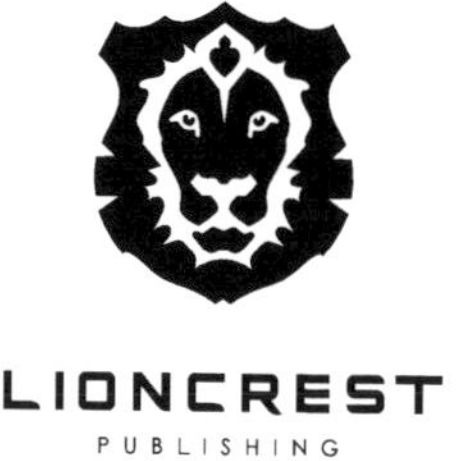

LIONCREST
PUBLISHING

I would like to dedicate this book to my family. My little buddy and beautiful wife Karen, my three loving children Gina Marie Maggi Crenshaw, Kimberly Dawn Maggi Dodson, Deno Taylor Maggi, and the seven precious grandchildren. I am getting ready to embark on my forty-second trip to Sierra Leone and have always had their full support without hesitation because they are so understanding of my dream. I love you all so much!

Contents

Foreword

By Neil Shulman, MD, Author of the novel Doc Hollywood and Associate Producer of the feature film Doc Hollywood starring Michael J. Fox

Darius Maggi is a REAL "Doc Hollywood." His pathway through a career as an obstetrician/gynecologist should enlighten all of those hoping to make the world a better place. His true humanitarian spirit of caring and dedicating his life to helping others goes beyond any novel I could ever write.

I had the pleasure of meeting Darius at a Global Health and Humanitarian Summit, which we initiated at Emory University in Atlanta, Georgia. There is no doubt that if everybody was like Darius, the world would be a place where future generations would truly live on a caring globe we could be proud of.

Darius' pathway through life as a practicing physician in Texas was such that he was psychologically tortured by a number of lawyers and patients who were not objective or self-critical. As a result, he quit practicing medicine in Texas and went to Africa to donate time and resources to help traumatized women in desperate need of medical care. Many of these women were psychologically and physically tortured because of lack of access to essential healthcare. For example, there were young women who needed a C-section because they were pregnant and the baby was too large to come out of the birth canal. Essential medical care was not available. Their babies died in utero and the medical consequences were so severe that these women experienced incredible pain and suffering. Dr. Maggi rolled up his sleeves and miraculously returned these women to a life worth living. He ultimately donated resources and attracted money, volunteer support, etc., so he could create the West Africa Fistula Foundation in 2004. The Foundation is located in Sierra Leone, West Africa where one in fourteen women were dying because of complications from pregnancy. Darius and his family, friends, co-workers, and philanthropists, come from a wide spectrum of backgrounds, and have united in hopes of changing the face of medicine in West Africa.

This true tale can inspire all of us to truly contribute to making the world a better place. I sincerely hope that the humanitarian messages in this book get out to the masses, for they have the power to positively impact every reader who picks it up. The psychologically gripping accounts of Darius's life story and his journey to find his humanitarian mission go way beyond what any fictional tale could accomplish. If Darius's message goes viral, then all of us can truly be proud to be members of the human species.

Introduction

I was probably seven or eight years old when I first remember hearing the word "basta." It was a common thread that connected my grandfather, my father, and me.

When my grandfather came to visit us from Chicago, he would say it to my mother when she fixed his breakfast—eggs, bacon, sausage, homemade biscuits and gravy, coffee—the works. He'd sit there at the kitchen table and eat very slowly, and my mother kept filling up his plate.

"Basta! Basta!" he'd say. "It's good! That's enough!"

He would say it to my workaholic dad to get him to slow down. "Deno! Basta! Basta! Enough! Enough is enough! Don't work so hard! You can only sleep in one bed. You can only wear one pair of shoes at a time. Your stomach will only hold so much! Basta!"

Of course, my dad still kept going full steam ahead.

Then, when I was practicing medicine and my dad saw

how hard I was working—being a workaholic ran in the family—he started saying it to me. "Basta! Darius! You don't need any more."

Of course, I still kept going full steam ahead.

I loved medicine. I enjoyed it so much I couldn't wait to get up in the morning and go to work. It was so gratifying, so much fun! I worked hours and hours every week, but I was full of energy. I'd wake up early and go all day. Being in obstetrics and gynecology, I would hardly sleep anyway. I was going, going, going.

Then I ran into obstacles—litigation—and I got really stressed. That's when my Dad said, "Basta! Enough! You've had enough of those folks. They're going to kill you. The stress is going to kill you. You've got to get out of medicine."

He was right. The stress was too much. But just the thought of leaving medicine was heartbreaking. I had worked so long and so hard to become a doctor, and I couldn't just walk away from a career I had put my heart and soul into. There had to be a way...

This is the story of how, in spite of what seemed to be the end of my career, my dream to continue the practice of medicine came true in the most unlikely of all places. As a little boy growing up in southeastern Oklahoma, I only wanted to be a doctor. I could never have imagined where this dream would take me. The adventure is far from over. In fact, it's just beginning.

My grandpa was from Italy. In 1905, he got on a ship by himself to come to the US via Ellis Island. He had $20 in his pocket. He was sixteen years old. He came to work in the coal mines. He never went to school, but he was very wise. It's phenomenal what I learned from him and from my dad. I still think of them and all the things I learned from them every day.

My grandpa and my dad were always very positive and, most of all, thankful that we had the opportunity to live in a free country. My dad used to say, "Son, freedom is not free."

I've been blessed to have people like them as my role models.

I always loved talking and listening to older people. I used to tell my kids, "If you hear enough of the same thing from older people, listen again because there's probably something to it. Your ears better perk up, and you'd better listen rather than talk and learn from what they're telling you." I remember a lot because I listened.

I'm extremely concerned about where our country is headed. It's all about me, me, me. It's all about selfies and the ego and selfishness that go with them. It drives me crazy. I think there's too much idleness among youngsters nowadays. For the most part, they don't have a good work ethic. They expect their first job out of college to be in upper management, with a salary to match. There is too much idleness—being bored is a common complaint. My dad used to say, "You weren't born knowing everything; that's why I've got to teach you. One thing I have to teach you is morals and ethics. The other thing is the value of a dollar. If I don't do that, I've failed you."

My granddaughter lives with my wife and me now, and I talk to her about the principles that have guided my life. I don't want her to have to go through some of the things that my grandfather went through, or my dad. Or me. If we can circumvent that, her life—and your life, too—can hopefully be even more productive and helpful to society.

I tell her about the Ten Commandments and the moral code. I tell her to be a good person and to tell the truth. I tell her to always do the right thing. That way, I say to her, you don't have to change anything or remember what you said. If you do something wrong, you will ultimately have to change it. That's what my dad used to say to me. "Son, it takes a lifetime to build a reputation, but you can lose it all in just a few minutes."

I don't want to be preachy, but I would love to see young people understand the importance of the basic values that I was taught. Hopefully, someone will read this book and get a sense of the true gratification and meaningfulness of life that I've been so fortunate to experience and will want the same thing.

I think a lot about the values I learned. I'm afraid they are being lost. That's what inspired me to write this book.

I'm not perfect. Obviously, in hindsight, there

are things that I would do differently. But I've had an extremely gratifying life.

Nothing is more meaningful to me than the work I do in Africa. I operate on fifty or so women each time I'm there. I remember one particular lady. She had undergone a hysterectomy a couple of months before I saw her. She came in with a huge mass in her pelvis. She was very poor and very malnourished. She was sick with fever. I examined her and found an abscess about the size of a cantaloupe. I took her to surgery that night, drained the abscess through the vagina, and put in a mushroom catheter. The next morning as I walked by her bed, she looked at me and said, "Doctor, thank you so much."

You couldn't give me $10 million and make me feel any better than that! Practicing medicine is not about the money. It's about relationships with people. That's why I founded the West Africa Fistula Foundation in Sierra Leone, because of the women whose lives we touched. They are extremely grateful for the work we're doing there. I'm extremely grateful for the opportunity to serve.

My belief system is based on the conviction that every person has a purpose in life. I believe it's not what we want out of life, but what life wants out of us and what we as individuals can contribute to society.

I'm not trying to tell anyone what to do in order to have a meaningful life. That's for each person to decide. I don't want to tell anyone that they've got to do this or that. It's up to every one of us to decide for ourselves and to discover what we can do to be of help.

I've always loved M. Scott Peck's book, *The Road Less Traveled*. I particularly like the following paragraph:

> *Life is not easy, and you have to accept that. A lot of people think life is just a joy ride, and it's not, especially if you're trying to make a difference in this world. You have to stand up for certain principles and your belief system and try to make the world a better place.*

I keep turning to Mitch Albom's books, *Tuesdays with Morrie* and *Have a Little Faith*. They have been very inspirational for me.

I keep a quote, compliments of Dr. Robert Kester, in my eyeglass case. I wear prescription eyeglasses when I operate, and I keep the quote in the case so that it's always handy. It reminds me that "evil will persist if good men do nothing."

Margaret Mead's famous quote is another favorite: "Never doubt that a small group of thoughtful, committed citizens can change the world; indeed, it's the only thing that ever has."

I grew up in the Assembly of God church and am a spiritual person. But I'd rather *see* a sermon than *hear* a sermon any day. In other words, instead of listening to someone preach to me about doing good and being right,

I'd rather see that person *do* some good instead of just talking about it. Actions speak louder than words. That's the way I try to live my life. I hope my actions will have a greater impact than the words I say.

This book is about the principles I learned from my grandfather and my father that have guided my life. It's about the importance of giving back and finding meaning in life. I hope it will inspire you to do what you can to help change the world.

I want this book to help people discover for themselves when enough is enough and to be able to say, like my grandpa did: "Basta! Basta!"

PART I

Oklahoma

A Grandfather's Wisdom

"When you're through changing, you're through."

They called my grandpa Madge in Oklahoma, but obviously it's supposed to be Maggi. His name was Arturo Maggi. He came to Wilburton when he was sixteen from an area near Bologna in Italy. The family homestead, sixty acres of farmland, is still there, though with different owners. My grandfather grew up working on the farm. He never went to school.

He came to the United States because times were tough in Italy. He'd already been to Germany in search of work when he was fourteen and ended up helping to build fortifications for Kaiser Wilhelm II, for which he earned four cents a day, or what a loaf of bread cost back then. He had heard there was good money to be had working in the coal mines around the small town of Wilburton. An Italian man named Mr. Antonelli sponsored him. Oklahoma became a state two years after my grandfather arrived. It was still Indian Territory then.

There were a lot of explosions in the coal mines in those days. One big one in Degnan, about three miles outside of Wilburton, killed more than100 men in 1920. I remember hearing my grandpa talk about it. I'm not sure exactly how long after that he decided to get out of mining, but soon he opened a grocery store on Main Street. The store was named Maggi and Son. I still have some old carbon receipts from the store with the name printed on the front.

Grandpa married a lady about fourteen years younger than he was. Her name was Teresa Torre. She, too, was born in Italy. They had three children: Ida, the oldest, then Joe, and my father Deno trailed behind.

Every Sunday night that I can remember, we called my grandpa in Chicago at 6:00 p.m. He had moved there when I was about eighteen months old to live with his sister. I'd hear my dad whistle from two blocks away when it was time to make the call, and I would run home. I always wanted to be there. We called him every Sunday until the day he died.

When my dad was six years old, his mother Teresa died at home in childbirth. Her mother, a domineering lady, came and got the two older children to take them back to Detroit with her. She wanted to take my dad, too, but he wouldn't go. He refused to leave my grandpa. He told me, "I cried, and I told her I'm not going. I'm staying with my dad." She left without him. It was just the two of them from then on, my dad and my grandpa.

They lived in a house that was adjacent to the store. I remember the store because it was still there when I was a young man. They walked twenty feet from their house, and they'd be at the grocery store. Just the two of them. They were so close. They had such a strong bond.

When my dad got drafted and left to go into the service, grandpa went with him to the train station. When my daddy was getting on the train, grandpa was lying on the ground crying. He lay there crying because he thought he might never see his son again. It hurt daddy so much to see his father so devastated that he didn't come home to visit before he was shipped overseas. He never took a leave. He knew that if he came home, it would upset grandpa too much when he had to leave again. He didn't come home until the war was completely over.

I'll never forget their house. In one room there was an old-fashioned ledger for receipts that was alphabetized, could fold up, and was spring-loaded. I remember finding an inch-thick wad of tickets with the balances brought forward. They were receipts from people who owed my grandfather money, hundreds and hundreds of dollars that he never collected. That's the way it was during the war. A lot of people couldn't pay for food, so grandpa let them have things on credit. He used to say, "Sometimes it makes you want to take your heart out and sit on it." He meant that people sometimes would take advantage of him because he was so good. But that's the way grandpa was.

He was very frugal, and he didn't waste anything. When they'd kill a hog, he used to say to my dad, "Now, Deno, the only thing we're going to lose is the squeal." Every bit of the rest of the pig they would eat or sell.

The only refrigeration they had was the Frigidaire in the grocery store. Because they didn't have a refrigerator in the house, they put some of their personal items, like butter, in the store refrigerator, to keep them fresh. People who came into the shop and saw the butter would want it. My grandfather, using his brain, would say, "Oh, *that* butter. Old lady Strong across the tracks made that butter." Well, old lady Strong was the filthiest lady in town, and nobody wanted to buy her butter. But she really didn't make it. He just told them that because he wanted to keep the butter for his son and himself.

My dad would send home all the money he earned every month, except 50 cents, which he kept to buy razor blades and soap. He did extra KP, too, so he would have more money to send home. When he came back from the Army, my grandfather pulled the rug back in the house, and there was $10,000! He had saved every red cent my dad had sent home. When my dad put the money in a bank account, the people at the bank told him that it was one-fourth of the entire capital of the bank!

Another example is when my dad was away during the war, and my grandfather had to shut the store down because he couldn't run it by himself. He didn't speak English well enough. In fact, when I got married and called to tell him, he said, "Happy New Year and all of that." I'll never forget him saying that. It was his way of congratulating me.

Grandpa was a wily guy. When he'd see the gypsies coming into the store, he would speak to my dad in Italian. He'd say, "Watch those gypsies, watch them. They're going to steal." Occasionally, they did steal, and my dad would have to chase them down the street to try to get back whatever it was they stole.

I remember grandpa would talk about the time the doctor came round to the house and pronounced his wife dead, after she had died in childbirth. This particular doctor was rather cold by nature. He ended up sending grandpa a bill, just for pronouncing his wife dead. That really hurt him. He would tell my dad, "I'm going to get even with him one day. I'll get even."

Later on, the doctor wanted to buy some cattle from

grandpa. My grandfather had a couple of pens with cattle that he kept on some land. When the doctor came to see the cattle, grandpa put the really good ones in front, in the first pen. The worst cattle he kept in the back. The doctor, naturally, wanted the good cattle, which were up front, and grandpa gave him a price though he didn't really want to sell them. Then the doctor asked, "What about those cattle in the back?" Grandpa replied, "Oh, those are my good cattle. I don't want to sell them." Of course, the doctor only wanted the good cattle. My grandpa appeared to be reluctant to sell him the really bad cattle. After the doctor left with the bad cattle, Grandpa said to my dad, "We're even now."

He was a big jokester, too. There was a gentleman, a black man, who would come to clean the septic tank for my grandfather. Every time he'd come, my grandfather would flip a coin, double or nothing. If the man won, my grandfather said he would pay him twice the fee. If my grandfather won, then he wouldn't have to pay him anything. That was the deal. They did it all the time.

The man would flip the coin and put it on the counter top. Then my grandfather would flip it and drop the coin on the floor, on purpose, so he could look up under the glass counter and tell whether the man's coin was heads or tails. He would always win. He never took any money, though. He was just teasing the guy—it was his way of joking. My grandfather always paid him. He would never cheat.

When the carnival came to town, there was one guy who ran a booth guessing people's weight. You had to pay if he got within so many pounds of your weight. My grandfather loved to trick him. He would wear his overcoat and stick a five-pound sledgehammer in each pocket. Then he'd hold his coat open while the guy frisked him to see if he had anything in his pants pockets. The guy never won. He always missed grandpa's weight. There was no television in those days, and grandpa's jokes were his entertainment.

When women came into the store and asked to use the restroom, grandpa made the logical assumption that they were tired and needed a place to rest. He would say, "I don't have any restrooms, but you can sit on the counter if you like."

Grandpa was about five feet five inches tall. He had sort of a heavy build and a little tummy on him. His hands had Dupuytren's contractures, a condition in which the fingers are permanently flexed. It involves the little finger and the ring finger and is more often found in Europeans. We don't know the cause of it. Some of it is hereditary, some of it is due to certain deficiencies. Both of his hands looked like a cup. If you shook hands with him, you would feel his thumb, and the other fingers would be nearly shut against the palm. I suspect that it may have been a consequence of his using a shovel when he was working in the coal mines when he was so young.

He always wore dark-colored dress pants and a short-sleeved shirt. I don't recall ever seeing him wear long sleeves. He buttoned his top button, at the collar, and his chin would jut out a little. He always had a hat on. He looked very young for his age.

Grandpa moved to Chicago to live with his sister Clara a year and a half after I was born. He worked for a natural gas company there, doing general maintenance. The only time I would see my grandfather was when he'd come home to Wilburton every summer for his annual visit, or those two or three times when we would go up there to see him.

He took the train to Oklahoma. The trip would take twenty hours or more. He'd have two suitcases. One was small, and it had just a few clothes in it. The other, a big old thing, would have a whole wheel of Asiago cheese in it, because we loved Asiago cheese on our spaghetti. He also brought pipe fittings from the gas company where he worked because he thought my dad might need them. It was hilarious.

My dad babied him during those visits. Grandpa was perfectly capable of taking care of himself. He was ambulatory, wasn't wheelchair bound, or at all weak. But my dad loved him so much that when he got up in the morning at about 4:30, he would go into grandpa's bedroom and wake him. He'd walk him to the bathroom, which was just across the hall, put him in the bathtub, and scrub him down from head to toe. Then he'd shave him and comb the two little hairs he had on his head. He'd put his underwear on him and powder all around. He'd powder him down like a baby and say, "I cleaned the monkey. I scrubbed the monkey." Then he put grandpa back in bed and let him sleep, and my daddy would go to work. He did that every time grandpa came to Wilburton in the summers, for at least fifteen years. My grandfather could have bathed himself, but he let my dad do it because he knew it was an expression of how much my dad loved him.

Finally, in the mid to late 1960s my dad talked grandpa into flying instead of taking the train. When he first walked down the steps of the plane in Tulsa, grandpa said to my dad, "You never get too old to learn." I heard him say that a million times.

I remember twice visiting my grandfather in Chicago. I went once with my mother, whom he called a "white fly" because he thought she was so rare, such a special woman. And once my dad went with us. It was the only vacation I ever remember him taking.

Grandpa went to live with his sister, Clara, because her husband had died, and she was alone. Aunt Clara made the best ravioli, tortellini, and spaghetti I've ever eaten. She lived in Highland Park and ran a boarding house. Down in the basement was a huge, long table. And she had a big stove where she cooked. She was a superb cook and rolled out dough by hand. Grandpa never went hungry!

And he liked his brew. He was good at making homemade beer and wine. He never sold what he made. Behind the grocery store in Oklahoma was a cellar that all the young kids in the neighborhood knew about. My grandfather would be working in the store when they'd come in. "Madge," they'd say, "there's a bad cloud coming up. We've got to go to the cellar. Give us the key." He gave them the key, but he found out later that what they really wanted was to stack bottles of beer and wine so they could reach them through the vent in the storm cellar. They put strings down the vent and brought up the beer and the wine.

I was very close to my grandfather. I was infatuated with him because my dad spoke so highly of him, even when he wasn't around. My grandpa told me to use my head, not my back, and he encouraged me to get an education, saying, "Put it in your head so you can take it with you."

Grandpa used to smoke a pipe. I loved the smell of the Prince Albert tobacco he used. It came in a little red tin. He'd flip up the lid and put the tobacco in his pipe. I remember the way he held it, with his middle finger due to the Dupuytren's contractures. He'd stuff the tobacco down a little bit, then light it. He'd puff on that pipe, and I loved smelling the smoke.

He loved America. He loved the freedom and was so appreciative. He was a simple person, very content, very laid back. My dad was hyper and high strung, but my grandfather was always relaxed.

He loved to walk up and down Main Street. He remembered all the people when he came back on his summer visits. He still had friendships and liked to visit with everyone on the street. One of his acquaintances was I. Yourman, a Jewish immigrant from Austria and owner of the jewelry store. Mr. Yourman also liked to tease my dad and say, “I came to America with more than you. I came with my clothes on.” Obviously, my dad was born naked.

I dreaded the day my grandfather would die. I knew it was going to tear my dad up. The love of my dad for his dad was unprecedented.

I remember once seeing grandpa have a transient ischemic attack, or TIA, which is a mini stroke, a short-lived deprivation of blood to the brain. It happens to people as a result of aging. I know exactly where he was sitting when it happened. I was chatting with him and all of a sudden he started going out. His speech was slurred, and he lost movement in his arm and foot. Fortunately, it resolved in five or ten minutes, and then he was back to normal.

He was eighty-six when he died from complications of an enlarged prostate. I was two days shy of turning twenty-two. One day I found out he was in hospital, and the next day he was dead. I remember my dad called me around 3:30 in the morning on November 19, 1970 and said that grandpa died. I was in my first year of medical school at the time. I was devastated. We buried him on my birthday, on November 21, in Oklahoma. They shipped his body back to Wilburton from Chicago, and we had a funeral. It was one of the saddest days of my life.

A Father's Work

"Always do the right thing. You don't have to change right, but you do have to change wrong."

While my grandfather was very laid back and content, my father was just the opposite. He was as hyper as a cat on a hot tin roof. He'd get up at 4:00 or 4:30 every morning and go to work. He loved life and every day he had a big smile on his face. He came home from the war on a Friday and went to work on Monday morning. That's how much of a workaholic he was. He didn't have a lazy bone in his body, and he didn't have much time for lazy people.

After all those years of working with my grandpa in the grocery store on Main Street, my dad's first job after the Army was for Mr. A. Lapp, a Jewish gentleman who owned a funeral home and a general merchandising store. It was a combined business: furniture, hardware, and funeral home all in one. My dad drove the hearse and picked up the dead bodies.

Then my dad ran the Magnolia service station on Main Street for a short time. Eventually, the name Magnolia was changed to Mobil. In 1949, Magnolia asked my dad to be a consignee, which meant that he bought gasoline on consignment. If he sold a gallon of gas, he might make two cents; if he sold 1,000 gallons he'd make $20, and if he didn't sell anything, he made nothing. His living was based on what he sold.

He had a warehouse and bought a little bobtail gas truck with a tank on the back. It held 978 gallons in five compartments: 303, 253, 107, 202, and 113. I know, because I filled them thousands of times. We put ethyl, or premium, in the 303 and regular in the rest. Then he hauled the gas to five filling stations in the area. In the late 1950s and early 1970s, when a lot of natural gas drilling was going on in the area, he hauled diesel, kerosene, and barrels of oil out to the drilling rigs.

He also bought and sold cattle. He purchased a farm from a lady he'd known since he was a little boy. She was a hairdresser. When her husband died, she sold the farm to my dad for $65 an acre, a total of $6,500 for 100 acres. She let him pay for it over a period of ten years. He'd planned for the annual payment well in advance in order to have enough money to make the payment, though he was always sweating it until the very end.

One thing my dad used to tell me was how much he missed his mother, and how it was so embarrassing for him when he went to school. The teacher would say, "Take this paper home and have your mother sign it." Daddy would break down when he said that. He told me how hard it was for him because he didn't have a mother, and how he always wished he did.

There were ladies in the community who knew his mother had died, and they always brought him food, cookies, and cakes. About three weeks before Christmas, until the day he died, my dad ordered thirty or forty boxes of cookies that came in oval-shaped cans with flowers on them. The Mistletoe Express truck backed up to my dad's warehouse where he kept the oil and gas, and unloaded all those boxes of canned cookies. On Christmas Eve, my dad would come home with grease all over him. Using a lot of soap, he washed up and put on clean clothes. Then, to show his appreciation, he took cookies to each woman who had given him things when he was a boy. Wherever they were, whether in their homes or in a nursing home, he never forgot them or their kindness when he was a little boy.

My dad went to high school in Wilburton but didn't graduate because he was too timid to stand up to recite poetry in front of the class. So the teacher wouldn't let him graduate. He never got his high school diploma, but he could recite poetry to the day he died. He never forgot anything, but he was very shy.

It was about three years after high school that my dad went off to the war. He left on a train from the station that was only half a block from his house. It was very hard for him because my grandfather lay down on the ground and cried.

Initially, my dad went to Louisiana, and then he went to Fort Benning in Georgia. After eight to ten months, he was shipped overseas where he stayed until the end of the war.

He told me he would never forget the invasion of Normandy. He was at the Utah Beach landing. The seas were very rough. They came in on a landing craft, lowered the ramp, and put a stake into the water to see how deep it was. If it was eight or ten feet, they had to back up and wait. Then they'd go back in and try again. He said he looked to either side of him and saw ramps go down and guys walking off the boats into the water and drowning.

He said he didn't take his boots off from May to September because they were constantly on the go. One July 4 they were surrounded. The Germans were bombarding them with artillery shells, but the shells fell short. He said it was because the French underground deliberately didn't put enough powder in the shells. The shells couldn't meet their maximum range, and, consequently, my dad and the others were saved.

Once he was driving a half-track, which is a vehicle with dozer tracks on the back part, when he ran over a mine and was blown off it. He had a concussion and shrapnel in his legs. He was hospitalized for a month. When he went back to the front line, a lot of guys he had been with had been killed. He thought his injury and the month recuperating in the hospital was why he made it. Otherwise, he probably would have been killed with the rest of his friends.

He told the Army not to tell his dad about his injury because he knew he'd come unglued if he heard my dad was in the hospital.

Daddy never got awarded the Purple Heart like he was supposed to. After he passed away, I found out that the building in St. Louis where the records were stored burned down. I was very frustrated that his injuries from service to the country he loved so dearly were never acknowledged.

I could see the scars from the shrapnel on his legs. He never got a pension or any kind of compensation for his injuries, and he didn't want any. He was simply happy to be alive.

My dad said that he would never forget Walter Chamliss, whom he had grown up with in Wilburton. He was in another battalion and found out where my dad was. He borrowed a jeep and drove over to see him. When my dad got back to Wilburton after the war, he found out that a sniper had killed his friend when he was on the way back to his battalion.

Dad remembered seeing General Patton with his pearl-handled guns, yelling, "Move those damn vehicles down the road and get busy." After Dad died, I was shocked to learn that he had helped free Holocaust victims. He'd also been at Berchtesgaden, Hitler's fancy house in the mountains. He took a bunch of pictures, some flags, and other stuff from the house and brought them home. I still have the Nazi flags. Other than that, he didn't talk much about the war, although whenever there was a thunder and lightning storm, he'd get scared and bolt out of bed.

About a year after my dad had returned home from the war, he married my mother. She was married previously to a man who was killed when he stepped on a land mine. They had a little girl, Janice. He was from Rochester, New York. His name was DiAntonio, and, not surprisingly with a name like that, he was a full-blooded Italian.

I was born in 1948, a couple of years after they were married. I was born in the town next to Wilburton where there was a hospital. My dad drove my mother there to have the baby. I also have a brother who is eight years younger than I am. He was born in 1956.

My dad worked hard to provide for his family. He had a lot of pride. My mother would starch his work clothes: khaki pants and blue or white shirt with the Mobil insignia—the flying red horse—on one side, and his name on the other. He left the house so neat and clean every morning. I thought we were rich because we had a house, but we were just living from paycheck to paycheck.

Behind my grandfather's store on Main Street and the house where my dad was born, there was a lot. Actually, it was across an alley that had once been an old railroad track. My dad bought that lot for back taxes. I still have the title. He used the money that he had sent home to my grandfather during the war and that my grandfather had stuck under the rug.

My dad built the house I grew up in on that lot. It was a beautiful rock house. My dad had rock hauled in from different parts of the state. At night when he got off work, he would put the rocks on the ground in the positions where he wanted them to go on the house. The rocks were beautiful and of many different colors. Before the house was finished, he ran out of money, and we had to live on the subfloors for two or three years until he could afford to put in hardwood floors and buy some furniture.

He bought his cars from a good friend who owned the Ford dealership in town. He bought a 1953 Ford, then a 1955 Ford, a 1957, and a 1959 Ford station wagon. Every two years he traded cars because he always wanted to have a safe car for my mother, even though he probably couldn't afford it. Then his friend sold the Ford agency, and daddy bought a 1962 Pontiac. After that, of all things, he bought a used 1965 Cadillac that an elderly lady had traded in. It had only a few miles on it. I said, "Oh, daddy, don't drive a Cadillac. It'll seem like we're trying to be something special in town." I didn't want to put on a front. My mother got mad at me and said, "Darius, your daddy works really hard. He's always wanted to have a Cadillac, and he wants to have a safe car for us." I never liked the Cadillac because I didn't want to pretend to be something I wasn't, and in my opinion that's what it conveyed.

I worked with my dad from the time I was old enough to crawl up into the truck. He had me filling tanks on the truck, which held 978 gallons. We would load that tank from one of the four 8,800-gallon storage tanks, which were about ten feet above the ground: one diesel, one premium or what we called ethyl, and two with regular gasoline because we sold so much more of that. It was all gravity flow. There was a little platform along the tank that I'd get up on. I put the spout in the tank and sat there to make sure it didn't run over. I was a little bitty tyke. I did that while daddy wrote the receipts.

We used a big stick to see how much fuel we had in the 8,800-gallon tanks. I'd scamper up the ladder, stake the tanks, and tell my dad how much was in each tank. Then he'd check the chart to find out approximately how much gasoline we had left. I helped my dad do all kinds of things like that. When we hauled gasoline to the filling stations, he had me figure out how much we had to charge them. We didn't use a calculator so I had to multiply it by hand every time. I've always been extremely good at math, thanks to doing that from a very young age.

When I graduated from eighth grade, my dad had me start working at a filling station owned by Troy Wagner for forty cents an hour, so I understood the value of a dollar. I worked six days a week, 10 hours a day. At the end of every week, the owner would tally the receipts to make sure we weren't off by a penny and pay me $22.60, once taxes were taken out. This was when my dad would come into my room at 5:00 a.m. and ask me if I was going to sleep my life away. He obviously felt he needed to instill a work ethic.

I will never forget one Sunday after church when my mother was preparing a special dinner, which consisted of a roast, mashed potatoes, green beans, salad, tea, and bread. My dad was complimenting her on how great the dinner was and she said, "Deno, that roast cost $5.00!" At that moment, I thought, "Oh my God! That roast cost $5.00 and I didn't even make that much in one day washing cars, filling the cars up with gas, and helping fix flats!" That really put everything in perspective. My dad always saved money and lived within his means. We never went out for Sunday dinner.

Daddy never cheated anyone out of anything. He got up at 4:30 a.m. to load the gasoline when it was still cold. That way it would expand during the day, and the station owner would get more gasoline. He tried to help the owners be successful and gave them credit. There was one guy who owned several businesses, and daddy used to go to the bank to borrow money so that he could cover his check. Almost every week, my dad would borrow $400 or $500 from the bank to pay for the guy's gasoline until he had the money. The guy always paid my dad, but it was delayed. Dad was always pro-station owner because he said, "Success breeds success." If they were successful, then they were going to help him be successful.

He was very astute as to what was going on. The only time he almost got cheated was when some guys from Shawnee came in and bought a lot of oil and wrote him a check. Daddy had pretty good-sized hands with calluses on them from all of his hard work. I'll never forget as long as I live seeing him write down the guy's license plate number on the palm of one of his big hands. Then he went into the office and wrote the number down on a big sheet of white paper that he kept on his desk. Of all things, it was a hot check, but since daddy had their license plate number, he got his money out of them. That was the only time he ever came close to losing any money.

When the energy crisis hit in 1973-74, he got out of the gas and oil business because it was no longer profitable, and he started a car wash. He hesitated at first because there was already a station in town, owned by a friend of his, that did a lot of car washing, but finally he decided to go ahead. He didn't have much of a choice because he wasn't able to sell gasoline any more. So he built a car wash and kept it until he died. I have it now. I ended up buying it from my dad. He also bought a small parcel of land close to town near the highway. We put a small trailer park with six slots on it, including sewer and water. We charged $20 a month for trailers to park there.

I'll always remember how my dad came home from work with grease all over him. We'd go upstairs, and he would get into the bathtub. He'd wallow in the tub and use Lava soap to scrub the grease off. I'd sit there on the toilet head and visit with him. He'd tell me about how he took baths in a number three wash tub when he was a kid because they didn't have running water. He'd say to me, "Thank God for running water. Son, we're so fortunate. We've got hot water, and we've got lights."

We didn't have air conditioning in the rock house, so in the summer we opened the windows at night and turned on the attic fan. My dad would go upstairs and turn on the fan at about 8:30 or 9:00 at night. My room was in the southeast corner of the house, and it had the nicest breeze. Then he'd get up about midnight and turn the fan off to save on electricity. When I brushed my teeth, he'd say to me, "Turn the water off. You're wasting water." During the day if I had a light on, he'd say, "Turn the lights off. You're burning daylight." He taught me from early childhood not to be wasteful.

One day he came home and showed me one of his highest commission checks. It was over $1,000 for the month, which was more than he usually made. My God! I couldn't believe it. Of course, what it didn't include were all the expenses my dad had for running the truck, keeping gas in it, insurance, and all the rest. But I thought we had gone to heaven. He made $1,000 a month!

I helped my dad a lot and went with him on Saturdays to deliver gasoline. He brainwashed me while we were driving down the road together in the truck. He kept telling me things he didn't want me to forget: Freedom is not free. Always do the right thing. Always tell the truth; that way you don't have to remember what you said.

We did everything we could to make a living. One evening after we'd finished working, we drove over to Fort Smith, Arkansas, and bought a house trailer. It cost $1,300. Dad had me go to the bank and talk to the vice-president about borrowing the money. He co-signed the loan. He wanted me to learn about responsibility at an early age. He also had me behind the wheel when I was young. When we were driving home that night from Fort Smith, daddy was so tired. He was weaving. I said, "Daddy, you're falling asleep." He said, "Then why don't you get over here and drive?" I took over the wheel and drove us home. I was all of twelve years old at the time.

We leased the house trailer to Sergeant Foster, the head of the ROTC program at the local college, for $50 a month. I'd go out there the first of every month, collect the rent, give him a receipt, and make the deposit at the bank. Then one winter, the pipes froze underneath the trailer. My dad and I went out in the middle of the night to wrap the pipes with tape to keep them from freezing. We did everything to make a living.

There was no such thing as an eight-hour workday. When I was about fourteen, we'd unload 50 to 75 barrels of oil, each weighing 450 pounds. We learned how to handle the barrels so we could roll them into the warehouse. Then we'd have to load them onto the back of the pickup to take them out to the oil rigs. Because there was a lot of manual labor involved with his work, Daddy got a cervical disc injury and had excruciating pain in his arms. He was in the hospital for a week, and I drove the truck. I would fill it up with gasoline, make deliveries to the stations, and unload it by myself—all before I went to school. I didn't even have a driver's license, but my dad had taught me how to drive early. I made deliveries to the station and unloaded by myself, generally late at night, so no one would notice. By the time I was ten or eleven, I was driving the pickup. When I was a teenager, I'd haul eight 55-gallon barrels of kerosene or diesel to the natural gas drilling rigs and hand pump the fuel into a larger tank at the well site. He never let me use an electric fuel pump because he wanted me to have a taste of hard labor so that I'd be sure to get an education.

On May 5, 1960, when I was twelve years old, we were eating chicken at about 6:30 in the evening when it started pouring rain. Then it started hailing. The hail was the size of a baseball. My dad and I walked out to the front of the house and saw Jim Cook, the state representative who lived across the street. Daddy started throwing hail balls at him. Then our neighbor, Mr. Walden, came out onto his porch and looked back to the southwest. He shouted, "Oh my God, Deno, there's a tornado!" I looked around and could see the tornado coming our way. Daddy said, "Darius, go tell your mother!"

I ran into the house and told my mother there was a tornado coming. She went to the back window to look. Then she ran to open the back screen door to go outside, but she couldn't open it because the pressure was so high. We all ran to the wrong end of the house, to the northeast corner instead of the southwest. My brother was about four then, and my sister was sixteen. We lay down and could hear the tornado coming our way. Like they say, it sounded like a huge freight train. It was headed from behind our house towards the front, and then it went over the hill. I could see debris flying all over the place. My dad and I went outside, and a guy was running down the street saying that the town had been destroyed.

My dad sent my mother, sister, and baby brother to a storm cellar three or four miles east of town, and he and I spent the night wandering through the town to see what was going on and to try to help people. We didn't know at the time that an F4 tornado had destroyed 15 square blocks, damaging or destroying 600 buildings, including 82 homes. Thirteen people died. That tornado was part of a monster storm system that raged May 4 to May 6 and spawned seventy-one confirmed tornadoes across Texas, Oklahoma, Arkansas, Kansas, Missouri, Iowa, Nebraska, Illinois, Alabama, and Mississippi.

About two blocks from our house was a nursing home. It was made of concrete blocks and had been completely leveled. We found an old man from the home wandering around, disoriented, with a suitcase in his hand. How it didn't kill him or any of the other people in the nursing home I have no idea.

There was no advanced storm warning systems then. No Doppler, no storm chasers who could send pictures directly to the meteorologist at the television station who could explain to viewers exactly what they were seeing in real time. There were no computers to predict a storm's path and pinpoint its exact location down to the street. About two hours later, people started yelling that another tornado was coming through. My dad pushed me down into a ditch and under a culvert. There was so much water, I thought I was going to drown. Everyone was yelling, "Here comes another one! Here comes another tornado!"

Trees were lying all across the roads. We walked down to Main Street and ran into Ben J. Thomas, a prominent businessman who owned a lumberyard and a hardware store. Blood was streaming down his face. The tornado had completely destroyed his huge brick building. I felt so helpless. My hometown of Wilburton, Oklahoma, had been a perfectly normal little town that morning with business as usual, and by midnight, it looked like a war zone, with death and destruction all around.

There were only three television networks at that time: ABC, NBC, and CBS—channels 2, 6, and 8 broadcast from Tulsa. Channel 10 was from Ada and broadcast a little bit of everything from the other networks. Each network sent reporters and camera crews to capture the damage on film and report it across the country.

Mr. Emroy Walden lived next door to us. He was from Mississippi. He was short, red-headed, and very fair skinned. He always wore a hat. His wife was obese and wasn't exactly the cleanest lady I'd ever seen. She regularly dipped Garrett's snuff. She kept a garden and raised chickens. I remember her grabbing the chickens and wringing their necks. She kept pigeons, too. He, on the other hand, was immaculate, always polite, and very pleasant.

Mr. Walden worked for the Rock Island Railroad. Every morning, wearing his blue overalls and a khaki shirt with a red and white hankie tied around his neck and carrying his lunch pail, he walked through our backyard, across the highway, and over to the railroad, which was a block away. He rode on one of the motorized four-wheeled carts used for going up and down the tracks, hand-driving spikes, and doing repairs. Sometimes I went with him, and he'd give me a piece of bubble gum they kept in a big compartment. I thought I'd died and gone to heaven.

I saw him come home at night. His shirt was drenched with sweat and his face was red. He could barely walk because he was worn out from working so hard. My dad would say, "Look at poor Mr. Walden. He's working for peanuts." Then he added, "But he's making a living."

Mr. Walden had two suits. Every Sunday, he put on either a blue or brown pinstripe suit and walked to the Methodist church. He always wore a brown and blue vest that went with both suits and a pocket watch on a gold chain. He always walked out of his house spotless to go to church. If the weather was really bad, he drove to the church in his 1951 navy Ford, which he kept parked in a small garage next to his house because it was too expensive to drive.

I was extremely close to him. After he got older, when I mowed our lawn, I mowed his lawn, too. He really appreciated it as he had the old reel type push mower. It took me no more than fifteen or twenty minutes.

When he retired, he loved to ride out to the farm with me and watch while I fed the cattle. But on Saturday afternoons when I asked him, "Mr. Walden, do you want to go feed with me?" he'd say, "Darius, if you don't mind, I'm just going to sit here." The real reason he didn't go was that wrestling was on TV. He'd come over to our house every Saturday afternoon around 4:30 to watch wrestling. He loved wrestling more than going to the farm. He thought it was the real McCoy. We laughed about how much he loved that fake wrestling.

One day when I was a freshman in college and had come home to have lunch, Mr. Walden walked out of his door saying, "Darius, I'm short of breath." I ran and got my mother. We put him in the car to take him to the hospital. He died of a heart attack before we got there.

Manuel Carter was a black man in town. He was a heavy drinker and lived in an eight-by-ten-foot shanty on the west side of town. The back of his house was propped up on rocks to be even with the dirt road. My daddy felt so sorry for him that he hired him for $4 a day to work at the farm.

Manuel and I would go out to the farm together and burn brush. We built a fence, using railroad ties as fence posts. First, we dug a hole two-and-a-half feet deep, put in a post, and tamped the dirt around it. We put the posts ten feet apart. Then we'd string seven strands of barbed wire. Manuel used to say, "Darius, you might ties it, but you can't beats it," meaning we'd make it straight as a string. My dad was very particular. To this day some of those ties are still there.

Sometimes Manuel would go with me to feed the cattle. We kept the feed in a fifty-five-gallon barrel. Sometimes when I didn't put the lid back on properly, I'd reach in and there'd be a dadgum possum in there with his mouth wide open, growling at me. Manuel said, "Let me have it." He'd get a pitchfork and kill the possum and say, "I'm going to have possum and sweet potatoes tonight."

When there was a heavy rain, the dirt roads flooded and big flatback turtles came out. "Darius, stop!" Manuel would say. Or if he wasn't with us, we'd grab some of the turtles, stick them in the back of the pickup, and drive by his house. He had a five-gallon bucket sitting on some rocks where he'd make a fire. "Put the turtle in that bucket," he said, "I'm going to have me some turtle soup."

Manuel was bad about drinking and got sick quite a bit. Daddy would tell Dr. Claxton, "Doc, if you take care of Manuel medically, I'll pay his hospital bills," which is what they did. When Manuel died, Daddy buried him and paid for his funeral. He got one of his suits, a shirt and tie, and put them on Manuel. There were about eight or nine of us at his funeral.

When I was a kid, every Sunday afternoon before we started eating, my dad took Manuel a plate of food. Then after Manuel and Mr. Walden passed away, we always took a plate of food to Mrs. Walden next door. Every Sunday. We didn't eat first and give them the leftovers. Daddy always said to my mother, "Go ahead and make a plate, and I'll take it to her." He did that every single Sunday.

My dad wasn't a well-educated person, but he had a lot of wisdom and a lot of common sense. He never yelled. He wasn't that way. But he was a disciplinarian, more with me than with my sister Janice, his stepdaughter. He was so nice to Janice and my mother. He was the most giving person in the world.

When my mother's first husband died in the war, she had received $10,000 from an insurance policy on him. My dad put it in a savings account for Janice. He was very emphatic that no one could touch the money. He said, "We're going to save that money for Janice to go to school."

When I was twelve and my sister was sixteen, I was in the seventh grade and she was in the eleventh. Janice was always very prim and proper; her hair was perfectly in place. She often ran late because she was so busy primping. She was voted the neatest person in her class.

I loved football, and I went to a game one Friday evening. When I came home, my mother told me that Janice had tried to kill herself. She had taken an overdose of Tylenol. They took her to Oklahoma City, and she was admitted to a private psychiatric hospital, where she stayed for several weeks.

She ended up with severe depression all through high school and for the rest of her life. Then she enrolled in a college, but she didn't stay long. She went to another college and didn't stay there, either. Eventually, my parents took her back to the psychiatric hospital in Oklahoma City, where they gave her electroshock therapy.

This went on for years. When I was in college in Norman, she was in Oklahoma City, and next thing I knew she had taken an overdose. I went up to Oklahoma City, put her over my shoulder, and carried her to the emergency room.

When I was in medical school in Oklahoma City, she'd come over to my place to visit. Once when she was visiting, she tried to kill herself with my .410 shotgun but ended up putting a hole in the wall. I asked her what was wrong. She said, "Darius, you just don't understand." She was in and out of mental institutions and psychiatric care for years. Her affect was very flat. I never saw her laugh or smile much again.

All of this was very expensive and stressful on everyone. Finally, when she was in her early 40s, she met a guy who was stationed at the air force base. His name was Jim Busko, and he was about seven years younger than she was. That was the best thing that had ever happened to Janice. They got married and ended up moving to Ohio. Then one day Jim called and said that Janice had tried to kill herself. She had taken an overdose. I was in practice then and was planning to fly up there, but my mother said, "No, I'll go see her." My mother flew to Ohio, spent a week with Janice, and came home. About three days later Jim called again and said Janice had hanged herself. She was fifty-two years old.

It nearly killed my mother and dad. My mother never did recover from it; she had so much guilt. My dad, bless his heart, didn't have a clue.

To this day there is not a single day that goes by that I don't think about my dad, ten or twenty times a day. I'm not obsessed, but I so much admire the type of person he was.

In the early 1980s, before the days of cell phones, I bought a portable mobile so I could be in touch with the hospital more easily, and every morning and evening I called my father on it. My dad would say "Son, you are spending so much on phone calls." I'd say, "One of these days, I'm not going to be able to call you." Sure enough, that day has come.

When I go back to Wilburton now, people say to me, "Oh, you're Deno's boy," because I look just like him. Once, an American Indian lady at Kentucky Fried Chicken came up to me and told me how much she loved my dad. She said that years ago when she was thinking about selling some of her oil and gas royalties, my dad told her not to do it because one day she may need the money. Of course, she would have sold them to him if he had wanted. "Now," she told me, "I'm living off that money." That's the kind of person my dad was. He wasn't about himself. He loved helping people.

I'll never forget my dad telling me that his school superintendent told him he would never amount to a hill of beans. Those were his exact words. My dad told me that story hundreds of times. Of course, my dad proved him wrong because he became, in my opinion, a very outstanding person.

My dad loved music. When he came home at night, he would turn on the radio or the record player. I never heard him sing. When he was on dialysis, my oldest daughter got married, and I saw him dance for the very first time in my life at her wedding. I have home movies of it. All that inhibition he had held inside him for so many years came out. He knew he didn't have long to live.

He died three months later at age seventh-nine, two days before the surprise birthday party I was planning for his eightieth birthday. I had invited around two hundred people. I chatted with him on the phone thirty minutes before he went outside and keeled over while he was moving the water hose.

PART II

A Doctor's Calling

Learning Medicine

"We are on this earth for a very short time. Be productive!"

I've always been the type of person who wants to fix things. When I was a kid riding in the truck with my father, and he'd tell me how much he missed his mother, I wanted to fix it. I didn't want to see women die from childbirth. I didn't want to feel the helplessness I felt on the night the tornado destroyed Wilburton and killed thirteen people. Then our neighbor, Mr. Walden, with whom I was very close, died in my mother's car. I saw my grandfather have a mini stroke and my sister's severe depression that led to her suicide. I suspect all these things, subliminally, inspired me to go into medicine. I wanted to be able to help.

Neither one of my parents had gone to college. My mother had taken some French classes for a short time, but that was all.

I did my first of year of college at Eastern Oklahoma State College, which was located in Wilburton. For my second year my uncle, my mother's brother, encouraged me to go to the University of Oklahoma because I wanted to be a physician. So I transferred there and spent the next three years in Norman.

When I first got there, I started playing intramural football. I was athletic and loved sports. I'd played football in junior high and high school. I was a quarterback and was spending all my time going to practice. We were undefeated, but by the first half of the first semester, I had eleven hours of Fs and four hours of Ds.

The dorms were old air force barracks. The rooms were small and primitive. Frank lived across the hall from me. He was a tall, skinny guy whose father had passed away. He didn't do well in high school, but he was bound and determined to go to medical school and become an eye doctor. He was very focused. His family didn't have money so he had to make good grades to get scholarships. He took twenty to twenty-three hours of classes every semester and made straight As.

Frank said, "Darius, you follow me, and you'll be okay."

We went to the library every Sunday through Thursday night, from 6:00 p.m. to midnight. We'd take a thirty-minute break at 9:00 to go to the student union and drink coffee. From then on, I was very disciplined. I made mostly As and brought my grade point way up.

Frank got into Tulane Medical School in New Orleans on a full scholarship, finished his residency at Tulane in Ophthalmology, and today he's an ophthalmologist.

I had always wanted to be a doctor. The only place I put in an application was the University of Oklahoma Medical School, which was about twenty miles north of Norman in Oklahoma City. If they asked you to come for an interview in November, it generally meant they were going to accept you on the spot. I received a letter to go for an interview Friday, November 14, the same day I was supposed to have a test at OU. I went to my physiology instructor and told him about it. He said, "We have a test that day, and if you don't show up, you'll get a zero." I'll never forget it; we were in the basement of a big classroom building. "In fact," he said, "I'll call them right now and reschedule your interview." I was so damned mad. He got on the phone and rescheduled my interview for December 26, the day after Christmas.

I thought I had a good chance of getting in because I had good recommendations and did well on my *MCAT* (*Medical College Admission Test*) scores. At Christmas, I went home and then drove up to Norman Christmas night. I got up very early the next morning because my interview was at 8:00 a.m., and I drove to Oklahoma City. The interviewer and I hit it off really well, but I was so disappointed when he said, "We're not accepting anyone right now because we have to go through all the other applications first."

In January, I was called up for a physical to go into the Army. This was during the time of the Vietnam War. I had my physical, number 156 in the lottery, and didn't know whether I was going to end up being drafted or going to medical school. This was particularly stressful because so many soldiers had died in Vietnam, many more were being sent there, and the political climate in this country was much different than it was in the early 1960s, when the United States first got involved in the war. Then on March 2, 1970, I was at home in my apartment when the mail arrived. I opened my mailbox and inside was a thick letter, which I took to be a good sign. The letter said that I had been accepted. I screamed and threw the letter into the air. I was thrilled! I was getting closer to making my dream of being a doctor a reality.

I did well in medical school. I didn't set the world on fire, but I did fine in all my courses.

The first two years we had basic sciences. Then we had exposure to clinical procedures. We worked in groups of sixteen students. A friend of mine, Jimmy Martin, was three or four years older than I was. Because my name was Maggi and his was Martin, we were in the same group.

Jimmy already knew his way around the medical center. On the weekends we would go to the emergency room with our short white coats on, and the interns and staff there would let us watch and see patients. Then they started letting us sew patients up.

As medical students, we were really excited about that. The first person I sewed up was a guy who had a gash over his eye. His wife had hit him. They'd been drinking. I was sewing him up when I went through tough skin and, boom, I went so deep I thought I'd got him in the eye! But I didn't. When he left, he said that he'd be sending his wife in next.

Jimmy had a master's degree in anatomy and was interested in seeing autopsies so we could learn more about anatomy. One day they were doing autopsies on two guys. One was much older and had been killed in an automobile accident. The other guy had died in jail. He had been an alcoholic and a smoker. I'll never forget how disgusting his liver and lungs were compared to the older guy who didn't smoke or drink. I saw what alcohol and smoking can do to the liver and lungs, how destructive they can be. That made a very big impression on me and influenced how I raised my children. I used to tell them that if beer, smoking, and pot would make them a better person, I'd be bringing home a case of beer, a carton of cigarettes, and marijuana every week. I remember in medical school Dr. Deckert, our psychiatric professor, used to say, "It's not the drink! It's the man! He would also say, "Do you drink because you're sick, or sick because you drink?" How profound are these words.

In our third and fourth years, we spent our time primarily in the hospital, rotating through all the services. We did internal medicine at the Veterans Administration (VA) hospital. For the most part, the nurses and the staff were lazy, maybe because they were employed by the government and knew they couldn't be fired. We did all the work. We filled out the X-ray forms and blood slips. We drew blood and took it to the lab. We got a lot of experience, and I became very good at drawing blood. We saw a lot of problems associated with alcohol. I remember having to stay in a single hospital room all night with an alcoholic going through withdrawal and having DTs (delirium tremens). He was screaming about his hallucinations—seeing spiders, snakes, you name it. I was there to make sure he didn't hurt himself. We were obviously not using restraints.

A lot of people at the VA hospital suffered from cardiac and respiratory arrests and were at high risk. I quickly became frustrated when we'd try to resuscitate them because so many of the interns and resident doctors couldn't intubate, put tube in the trachea. It's very important to get a tube into a high-risk patient so that they'll be able to breathe.

After I finished the internal medicine rotation, I

changed my schedule and went to see Dr. Carmack, the head of the anesthesia department. I told him that I wanted to learn to intubate. He was very nice and took me under his wing, saying that if I came to work with him, he'd teach me everything I needed to know. He said that by the time I left, I'd be very proficient. I spent five more weeks at the VA hospital, and all I did was go from room to room in the surgical suite putting tubes in patients who were being anesthetized. I put in endotracheal tubes. I put in nasotracheal tubes. I even intubated babies. I put in hundreds of tubes during those five weeks. I got to where I felt very comfortable intubating patients. Today, generally, only doctors who are going into anesthesia as a specialty learn how to intubate.

I was good at intubating because I wanted to fix things. I also got really good at doing spinal blocks. A lot of the veterans had prostate problems and needed surgery, which is generally done under spinal block anesthesia. You put a needle in the patient's spine, and they are numb only from the waist down. I gave hundreds of spinal blocks and became very confident.

In my third year when I went through the surgery rotation, one of the medical students didn't show up for an operation. They asked for someone to replace him, and I volunteered. It was a ten-hour surgery, a Whipple procedure for treating cancer of the pancreas. It normally doesn't take that long, but the resident doctors who were doing the surgery were still learning. I was the low man on the totem pole. I stood there for eight to ten hours and was grilled by the intern and resident about anatomy. Since I hadn't been assigned the case, they went relatively easy on me. At about 3:00 p.m., the chief surgical resident stuck a Hershey bar under my mask because I hadn't taken a break all day. That was my first surgical patient. He was a very sick man, and I had to give him fluids, monitor his electrolytes, and keep a close eye on him for several weeks. I learned a lot through that experience.

Another one of my early surgical patients was a sheriff from Tuttle, Oklahoma, who needed open heart surgery for a heart valve replacement. He had been assigned to me, and we became very close. He and I would shoot the breeze all the time. One morning he was scheduled to go into surgery at 6:00 a.m. I arrived plenty early, but they had already taken him into the operating room. He ended up dying on the table. It broke my heart, and when I got home, I broke down and cried.

I hated obstetrics when I was in medical school because the head of the department was a horse's ass. He was the most egotistical guy I'd ever met. I couldn't stand him because he was such a prima donna. He screamed and yelled at people all the time. He was extremely cocky, very hot-tempered, and narcissistic. It was his way or the highway. Despite all that, I ended up taking an elective rotation of obstetrics in my fourth year.

It was a ten-week rotation. One of my fellow medical students was seven or eight years older than I was. His wife was pregnant and had delivered her baby in a private hospital in the northwest part of town. He went there to be with his wife and missed a day in the hospital. Because of that, the head of the department flunked him for the whole year. He had to repeat the entire year because he had missed only one day.

Another incident occurred when the three of us on the obstetric rotation were supposed to attend a cancer conference. I was there, and the head of the department asked me where the other two were. I told him that I didn't know. He left the conference, walked down to the hospital's public cafeteria, and found them there. He screamed and cussed at them in front of everyone and told them to get back upstairs to the conference. Unfortunately, he had a lot of power because he was very high up in the American College of Obstetrics and Gynecology. That didn't make any difference to me. I still didn't respect him. Bottom line was he turned me off going into obstetrics and gynecology.

I remember the first baby I delivered. The mother was a stout lady. It was her sixth or seventh baby. I had been by her bedside all night, and she said to me, "You just sit there, and I'll tell you when the baby's coming. I'll just push it out." And, boy, did she! It was a very easy delivery.

Another lady who was very obese came into the hospital in labor. She swore up and down that she hadn't had a clue that she was pregnant. While she was lying on the couch watching TV, her water broke. She came in and delivered a baby.

Before I finished my fourth year, I moved to Tulsa to do a rotation in cardiology, which I really enjoyed. I worked with three doctors, Neal, Zoller, and Raines, who had a huge practice. They had thirty or forty patients in the hospital at all times. I worked hard and loved it. I saw lots of people with heart attacks, which I found very intriguing. Heart attacks then were much more prevalent in men than in women, because more men smoked. However, the incidence in women has increased, because more women are smoking. Now, heart disease is the number one cause of death in both men and women.

On July 1, I started my internship. I'd always wanted to be a primary care doctor when I was in medical school because there had been a lack of family doctors in my hometown. So I did my internship in family practice at a private hospital in Tulsa. There were seven of us interns. We were the last group to be able to do a rotating internship. We spent time working in all the specialties: internal medicine, general surgery, pediatrics, obstetrics and gynecology, and more. Today, most graduates go immediately into a specialty. Rotating internships are pretty much gone in most hospitals. I also did a rotation in orthopedics and dermatology, because I wanted a full range of experience.

A lot of the time, we were the only doctors at night in the 600-bed hospital where I did my rotating internship. If a patient came into the emergency room in the middle of the night, we got up. Or we'd have to run down to the ward to take care of a patient. I was able to put my intubating skill to good use. I could intubate almost anyone. I was also good at starting IVs. I learned to put in subclavians, which is another way of inserting an IV under the clavicle if someone is hemorrhaging.

One time, a young man who was an alcoholic came in. He was throwing up blood and went into shock. He did not have a blood pressure, and his pulse was very weak. We put his head down and feet up, and I was able to get a large catheter in his subclavian vein to transfuse him with fluids. Fortunately, he lived. This gave me a lot of confidence and made me happy that I knew how to do this.

When I worked in the emergency room, lots of women came in with premature deliveries. Neonatal Intensive Care Units weren't common at the time. I'll never forget one baby born at around thirty-two weeks who had respiratory distress syndrome. A very nice pediatric cardiologist, Dr. Charles Cooper, was there to help me. We intubated the baby to try to help it breathe, but we didn't have a pediatric respirator. There was nothing else we could do because we didn't have the equipment we needed, and the baby died. Today, that baby would have had a very good chance of making it.

At the end of my internship, I joined a private practice in Durant, a town in southern Oklahoma. I did everything there. I took care of heart attacks. I delivered babies. I worked in the emergency room. Once a guy came in after a horse fell on him and crushed his chest. I intubated him immediately. Suddenly it was hard to squeeze the bag, which meant his lung was unable to expand because of pressure from air in the chest cavity (better known as a tension pneumothorax). The treatment is to immediately insert a chest tube to release the air. Because I didn't know which side of the chest was affected, I put tubes on both sides. That relieved the pressure on his lung, and it could expand normally.

A little boy about ten years old came in. He had been climbing a rope in gym class and fell to the ground, convulsing. I intubated him and started an IV to sedate him. Then I turned him over and did a spinal tap. When I got blood, I thought he must have bleeding in the brain and sent him immediately to a neurosurgeon who did an angiogram. Turns out he had an aneurysm, which is extremely uncommon in children. Thankfully, he did well.

Then there was the president of an oil company who was waterskiing while drunk at Lake Texoma. He had a fracture dislocation of his shoulder. There was no pulse in his arm, which meant the break had compromised his blood vessels. He would lose his arm if the fracture wasn't reduced. I first gave him medicine to relax his arm muscles, and then I was able to reduce the fracture and refer him to an orthopedic surgeon.

I saw people with heart attacks and many other things, and I quickly realized that I needed more training. I thought about going into pediatrics, which I loved because children could be so sick one minute you thought they might die, and then twenty-four hours later, they'd be running around all over the place! I also considered obstetrics and gynecology, which usually ended in a happy event. There'd be an end point, a result—after nine months, a baby is born.

I called my friend, the ophthalmologist who had gone to Tulane School of Medicine in New Orleans, and asked him about the obstetrics/gynecology program at Charity Hospital, which was the teaching hospital associated with Tulane. He told me that I should come down there. He said if a third-year medical student could deliver as many babies as he wanted, there was no telling what I'd be able to do as a resident.

I jumped on a plane (my first commercial flight) and went down to check it out. I really liked what I saw. The hospital had an extremely high volume of patients. They did as many as 12,000 deliveries a year, and there weren't enough residents because not many residents wanted to work that hard. They accepted me and in late December 1975, I moved to New Orleans with my wife and our one-month-old baby girl. On my first day, January 1, we had twenty-one deliveries!

I saw everything at Charity Hospital because of the phenomenal volume, everything in the obstetrical book: women with high blood pressure, women coming in convulsing, women who were bleeding, numerous sets of twins (we had one resident who delivered two sets of conjoined twins), abdominal pregnancies, women with sickle cell disease, kidney failure, or severe anemia, and pregnant women with tumors. I saw everything imaginable.

The first four to five months I was on obstetrics service, and I worked around 140 hours a week. When I was on call, I never slept because there were so many deliveries and we were so shorthanded.

I was in my element. I can read about something all day long and not be good at it. But if I see it and do it, I'll never forget it. An example is abruptio placentae, which is when the placenta separates prematurely. In one month we had thirty cases of it, which is unheard of. We saw placenta previa, which happens when the placenta covers the opening of the cervix. We saw ruptured uteruses. Women came in with sky-high blood pressure due to preeclampsia. We saw women who were blind because of severe toxemia.

I loved it because I was getting so much experience, and I wanted to be good at what I did. I knew that when I went out to practice on my own again, there would be very few things that I hadn't already seen at least several times in my residency.

Then I did the gynecology rotation and saw women

with miscarriages and tubal pregnancies—not just one a night, but three or four. Once I treated six women with miscarriages in one night. Women came in bleeding from very advanced cervical cancer, whom we often had to send home to die because there was nothing we could do for them, even with a special ward for advanced cancer patients. Women came in very ill with big tubal ovarian abscesses due to pelvic inflammatory disease. Women who had had an abortion would come in septic, running a high fever. Every day I had all these different types of cases over and over again.

Charity Hospital, the second oldest hospital in the United States after Bellevue in New York City, had 2,680 beds, all for indigent patients. Doctors doing general surgery saw gunshot wounds, automobile accidents, and bleeding ulcers. You name it, they saw it. It was the same in pediatrics, orthopedics, and internal medicine—strokes, heart attacks, kidney failure. Whoever trained at Charity Hospital got a phenomenal amount of practical experience. We may not have been able to quote the latest journal article but we had pretty much had seen it all.

After six or eight weeks, I started doing C-sections. After eight or nine months, I was teaching how to do a C-section. It was see one, do one, teach one. Everyone wanted to teach the person under them so that person could take up some of the slack. We were all trying to help each other because we were so short staffed. Generally, the residents taught us, not the staff doctors, who were rarely there.

What you didn't ever want to do was to lose a patient, because then you risked getting kicked out by the head of the department. We prided ourselves in truly taking care of the patient. I will never forget one of our sickest patients who postoperatively had to go to the ICU. We as the residents spent the night with that patient in the ICU until she was moved back to the ward.

While I was at Charity, we lost only one patient. She was the daughter of one of the security staff, whom we all liked a lot. She came in convulsing from toxemia, and we did an emergency C-section. Postoperatively, the woman developed postpartum psychosis and split her incision open. When one of my fellow residents took her back into surgery to sew the incision up again, she aspirated and died, which was an anesthetic death. The resident went into severe depression, and to this day, he doesn't like to talk about it.

• • •

A young thirteen-year-old African-American girl came in with really high blood pressure. I saw a lot of young girls who were pregnant. I was treating the blood pressure and giving her medicine not to convulse, and I was trying to induce labor to get her to deliver, which is standard treatment for preeclampsia, or toxemia pregnancy. I kept telling the resident over me, "I don't think she's going to deliver. I think we're going to have to do a C-section." And he kept saying no, that I should keep giving her medicine and try to get her delivered. Finally, I took her in for delivery, and he told me to use forceps. So I gave her a spinal block and put forceps on. She started hemorrhaging terribly because her placenta had separated prematurely. Fortunately, I got a live baby, but she kept hemorrhaging. I thought she was going to die. She went into what we call DIC, or disseminated intravascular coagulation, which is a bleeding problem. I had already asked the medical student who was assisting me to get blood ready, and we managed to save her life, but it was very close.

Another patient ruptured an ovarian vein, an extremely rare occurrence, and had gone into shock a few hours after she delivered. We saved her, too. The doctor over me at the time came in to check on the situation and insisted, once the patient was stable, that I have an X-ray taken of her abdomen to make sure we did not leave a sponge or instrument in the abdomen because thing were really hectic at the time. I taped a clamp to the lady's back, which, of course, showed up on the X-ray. The supervising doctor had a fit, thinking we would have to re-operate, but then he realized it was joke and the source of some much-needed laughter to relieve all the tension we had been under.

In my second year, they sent me out as chief resident in a rural charity hospital. Obviously, my superiors liked what I was doing. I was put in charge of a first-year resident, an intern, and a couple of medical students. This hospital also had a very high volume of patients, including 300 to 400 deliveries a month.

We had a lady who came in, and an intern had given her a spinal block in order to put forceps on the baby. The spinal block went too high and affected her respiration, which caused her to have respiratory and cardiac arrest. I was in the chief resident's house at the time. They called me at 2:00 a.m. to come right over. I ran out of the house while pulling on my scrubs. When I got to the ward, the patient was not breathing and had no heartbeat. I immediately intubated her and injected her heart with adrenaline. Fortunately, she responded with a good heart rate, and her blood pressure returned to normal. After she was stable, I put her legs in the stirrups, put forceps on the baby, and delivered a beautiful, healthy baby. After several hours and checking in with staff in New Orleans who had told me to do the best I could under the circumstances, I took her off the respirator. When she woke up, she couldn't see my fingers. She was blind! I thought this was due to cerebral edema (swelling of the brain) and gave her steroids to help with the swelling. Four hours later she could see again! The next day she and her baby checked out of the hospital, and both did very well.

Then there was the lady who came in with convulsions due to toxemia and pulmonary edema due to heart failure. The build-up of fluids in her lungs made it extremely difficult to breathe. Because she was convulsing, I was unable to put a tube through her mouth and had to do a blind intubation by putting a tube through her nose and into the trachea to establish an airway. We ended up delivering the baby under local anesthesia because of the severity of her condition. After a few weeks in the hospital, both she and baby were fine.

It was a very stressful time because I was the person in charge. I was only twenty-seven years old. I had been given an incredible amount of responsibility. That would never happen today. Now, professors are in the room with residents all of the time, even during a normal vaginal delivery. That's due to the fear of litigation.

All that experience built up my confidence. During my years of residency, I did hundreds of vaginal hysterectomies. Now doctors graduating from a residency program may have done only six or seven. Of course, just because I have done hundreds doesn't mean that I won't have any problems or complications, but the likelihood of my being able to take care of something is much greater if I've had experience doing 300 or 400 hysterectomies versus doing only half a dozen.

After my residency, I moved back to Durant and started practicing on my own. I was on call every night because of the lack of what I considered to be good enough back-up coverage. For twenty months, I took calls every single night by myself. My wife and I had two children at the time. It was an untenable situation. I decided to move across the Red River to Denison, Texas, which had a much larger hospital with an excellent reputation and nearly every specialty, other than open heart and transplant surgery. That was very unusual for a town of its size.

During the time of my internship before starting a practice, when I was on orthopedic rotation, I encountered one of the best clinicians I've ever known in my life. His name was Dr. Vosberg. He had a big impact on me. I was very impressed by the way he treated people. He was an orthopedist and practiced medicine very, very conservatively. He was a tall guy, a basketball player for years, and had a very deep voice. He'd see a person with back pain and say, "Now, Myrtle, you go home and do this or that. I'll see you back here in two months. If you get worse, come on in, but let's see how you do." I'd say he treated 80% of his patients like that, conservatively. And he got great results. If they didn't get better, he'd intervene, but surgery was always the last resort. The neat thing was he was so dadgum busy because everyone knew he wasn't knife-happy. He wouldn't operate on everybody who walked through the door.

When I went started practicing medicine on my own and began a private practice, I used Dr. Vosburg's approach. The word got around that I wasn't going to operate on anyone unless they needed it. I was swamped.

But I also started to have a life again in Denison. I rotated calls with another OB-GYN and could take off a weekend or a night during the week.

For me, having a big practice wasn't about making more money. The money was there and I was making a good living, but I was also able to give so much away. I wouldn't charge many people at all. And I loved to play jokes. I always tried to use humor to help break the ice. I had inherited my grandpa's sense of humor and love of playing jokes on people.

When I was working in Durant, I had a nurse who was just as sweet as she could be. She said to me, "Doctor, I need a Pap smear, but I'm embarrassed. If you don't mind, I'm going to put Burt Reynolds on the ceiling." So she put a picture of Burt Reynolds on the ceiling of the exam room, and I did her Pap smear. "Well, that wasn't so bad," she said afterwards. She forgot to take the picture down, and when the next patient came in, she saw Burt Reynolds on the ceiling and loved it. Soon word got around that there was a photo of Burt Reynolds in the exam room. Next thing I knew, people were getting frustrated if there wasn't picture of a movie star on the ceiling, and they'd put another one up. Everyone loved it because it took their minds off the exam.

Also in Durant, I had a lady whose mother was very close to her and wanted to see her daughter's delivery. There were rules that family couldn't be in the delivery suite, but it was the middle of the night when her daughter started delivering. So I told the mother to come on in. We were in an old surgical suite, and she stood by the scrub sink, looking through the window into the delivery room. I delivered the baby and held it up for the grandmother to see. She was probably seventy years old and was clapping and so happy. Then I clamped and cut the cord, put the baby on the mama's lap, and acted like I was reaching back up to deliver the placenta. I turned back around to the grandmother and put two fingers up, informing her that there were two babies. When I looked back again, she wasn't there. When I ran out to find her, she had passed out and was lying flat on the floor. I feared I had killed that lady. I thought that she'd probably had a heart attack, or if not, when she passed out, she had hit her head on the scrub sink. Fortunately, she was fine, and we laughed about it together forever.

Later, I started letting husbands deliver the baby about 90% of the time. When husbands came in while I was examining their wives, they often felt somewhat uncomfortable. So about the time the baby was coming, I'd tell the husbands to put on a gown and I'd say that one of their buddies had done the same thing, so then they'd want to do it, too. After a while, they loosened up and let me put a gown and gloves on them. Of course, the women loved it. They wanted their husbands in the delivery room with them. Then when the baby's head started coming out, and

I'd say to the husband, "Now, come down here and help me hold the head." The husband would hold the head down, and then I'd say, "OK, now just pull a little bit on the head." Then I'd stand back and the next thing they knew, they had delivered the baby. They were so elated and proud of themselves. They had forgotten all about their hesitations and concerns, and it was good for their bonding with the newborn.

Sometimes, I would hand the husband a clamp for clamping the umbilical cord, but I wouldn't give him the go-ahead. When I saw that he was clamping the cord, I would turn my head away and pretend that I hadn't seen anything. When I heard the sound of the clamp, I said, "Now don't clamp the cord until I tell you to," and he'd want to pull the clamp off. Then I said, "Well, I'm sorry if the baby doesn't make As in school. It's not my fault. You clamped the cord too soon." Of course, he hadn't. I was just teasing the guy. They all loved the humor because it helped them relax.

The husbands became very comfortable with me, a male, taking care of their wives. I built a rapport with all of them. I got to be good friends with many of my patients and their spouses. It wasn't just one person who was my patient; the entire family was part of being the patient.

Recently, I ran into a guy in a restaurant who came up to me and said, "I'll never forget how you helped me deliver my baby." His baby was born with Down syndrome.

He said, "I love that kid. It means so much to me to have been able to deliver my son. I'll never forget it."

One lady who was having a baby was rather stout, and her husband was a tall, skinny guy. I was doing a C-section on her, and he was sitting next to the anesthesiologist. Every once in a while he'd peek over the drapes a little to see what was happening. About the time I was taking the baby out and there was blood, I heard an awful racket. He had fallen back against the stainless steel shelving that was filled with supplies for the operating room. His wife looked over at him and said, "Get up, you wimp. I'm having this baby. Not you." It was so funny. To this day, I call him a wimp. It's relationships like that and the friendships you build that make the difference. It's one of the best ways to take the anxiety out of medicine.

When the wife of a good friend of mine was in labor with their third baby, my friend had asked to borrow my video camera, which I took to the hospital with me. He needed to take his young daughter and son to the babysitter's so I said that I'd come by to pick up his wife and take her to the hospital. By the time he got to the hospital, she was already in early labor, so he went to get the movie camera. I don't know where in the world he went, but he was gone for a very long time. When he finally walked in, I said, "You missed the delivery." He turned white as a sheet and broke out in a sweat. He knew that his wife would give him holy hell if he missed that delivery. I was kidding him, of course.

Once I switched a baby. An elderly lady, close to eighty years old, had a huge mass in her abdomen and looked like she was ten months pregnant. Though I was 99% sure the situation was benign, I operated on her. Sure enough, it was a non-malignant growth. I went to check on her during postoperative rounds, and her family was with her. I'd already told her kids, who were probably in their 50s, that I felt it was benign, though we always send a specimen off to the lab to know for certain. That night, the lady was still apprehensive, so I walked into the nursery and picked up a baby. I went back into my patient's room and said, "Mary, this is what I got out of you. I don't know how you're going to explain that to your kids!" Her family about rolled on the floor from laughing so hard, and she got tickled, too. It broke the anxiety and took their minds off of cancer.

Another time I went to visit a patient, a single mom, just after she had just delivered a baby girl. When I went into her room, she was bawling. "What's going on here?" I asked. She replied that she had wanted a boy and was bawling away. I said, "Look how healthy this pretty little girl is."

"I don't care," she said, "I wanted a boy."

"Okay," I said to her, "let me have this baby. I'll be back."

I took the baby and went to the nursery, pulled its diaper down, and put in a rubber nipple. I put the diaper back on, went back to the mom about twenty minutes later, and said, "I did a sex change. Here's your boy."

"You did what?" she said.

"I did a sex change on the baby. Just look." And I pulled the diaper back, and there was the nipple sticking up.

Then there's the story of Roxanne, when she was having her first baby. Roxanne's mother was a patient of mine, too. Roxanne thought she was in labor, and she and her mother drove from Durant, across the Red River, to see me in Denison. At about 11:00 a.m. I examined her and told her that she might be in early labor, but because it was her first baby, I told her to go out to the mall with her mother, walk around, come back in a couple of hours, and I would check her again.

They walked around the mall for a while and came back. I checked her, and things had changed. So I sent her to the hospital. When I checked again later, Roxanne was in early labor. Her mother, Betty, wanted to call the family in Oklahoma to tell them the news, but the phones were out that day. So she had to drive across the river. It took her about an hour and a half to get over there and back. For some reason, Roxanne started having really hard contractions and delivered the baby before Betty got back, which was wonderful as it was her first pregnancy.

I said to Roxanne, "When your mother gets back, we're going to have some fun." I told her to stick a pillow on top of her tummy. I put a cover over her and hooked the fetal monitor back up as if we were listening to the baby's heartbeats.

When Betty came in, I said, "She's not in labor. I thought she was, but she's not. I'm going to send her home."

Betty said, "Oh no, I want a baby today."

I repeated, "Betty, I'm trying to tell you she's not in labor. This is her first baby." Then I said, "Okay, if you want a baby," and went into the nursery and got the baby Roxanne had just delivered. I handed the baby to Betty and said, "Here, take this baby."

"I don't want that baby!" Betty exclaimed.

Then I asked Tex, Roxanne's husband, and Roxanne what they thought about Betty not wanting the baby.

Later, when I told Betty that Roxanne really had delivered the baby, she started boo-hooing and was so excited. It was a lot of good fun.

When you're dealing with a pregnant lady and go in with a frown on your face or a concerned look, you're going to cause a lot of apprehension. The mental aspect is so important when treating patients. That's why I try to use humor a lot.

When I was in medical school, I had one professor for all four years who was absolutely superb. He was outstanding. He was a psychiatrist and probably one of the smartest men I've ever known in my life.

He used to tell us, "If you do not listen to the patient and take a good history, you have failed the patient and yourself. You, as a generalist, will find out that 75% of all people will have an underlying psychogenic cause for why they've come to see you." He said, "In ten years' time, you'll call me and tell me how right I was." I did call my professor ten years later and said, "Gordon, you were right on!"

And that's why I had an extremely successful practice. I listened. I had more than 15,000 patients over the years. I had such a phenomenal following because I listened to every one of them. I took note of their stresses and depressions and tied that into treating the whole person, rather than just treating their uterus or their vagina or their menstrual period.

I always try to be very positive, very uplifting. I teased women about having twins or said, "I sure hope this baby doesn't look like your husband, because if it does, it's sure going to be ugly."

I always tried to compliment a lady and was honest about it. I know that a lot of pregnant women don't feel good about how they look especially near the end of pregnancy, and I felt they needed a little boost of encouragement. I always tried to be very positive because I know giving birth is a life-changing event for a woman. Having a baby should be wonderful for everyone involved.

I operated on a thirteen-year-old girl when I was in the outlying hospital during my residency. She came into the emergency room with severe cyclical pelvic pain. Because of her age, I examined her under anesthesia and saw that the vagina was blocked with what we call a transverse vaginal septum, a condition she was born with. This thick window of tissue was located about halfway up her vagina and kept her menstrual period from exiting her body. It built up month after month and created a bulge in her rectum. I drained the blockage through the rectum and later took her back to surgery and resected the septum, taking care to avoid the bladder and urethra. Several years later when I was in practice, I received a huge envelope in the mail with a copy of the birth certificate of the baby she had recently had. She'd named him after me.

There are a number of little boys named Darius down in New Orleans now, and in Oklahoma, too.

The Dark Side of Medicine

"Call an ace an ace, and a spade a spade!"

I got out of medicine when I was hitting my prime as a physician. I was nearly fifty years old. I prided myself on all the experience I had and on not doing things unnecessarily.

An example is the case of a woman whose husband I'd grown up with who was also my patient. I had delivered her second baby, but hadn't been there when her first child was born. She came to see me with a big ovarian cyst. It was a little larger than an orange.

I looked at her and said that I was 99% sure it was

benign. I told her I didn't think we needed to do a lot of expensive tests. I'd seen cysts like that many, many times. I told her to come back in three months for a recheck and that if she had any pain or problems before then to come see me. Three months later she came back, and the cyst was gone. I saved her and her insurance company thousands of dollars.

I can guarantee that 98% of doctors today would have done an ultrasound, or a CT scan, or more, which costs patients a huge amount of money and creates a lot of apprehension and anxiety. Why do that? Today, most doctors do it because, number one, they're afraid of getting sued, and number two, they don't have the experience.

When I was doing general practice medicine and working in the emergency room before I went into my specialty, kids would come in all the time with head injuries from falling. I would do a complete neurological examination on them and if everything was normal, charge $35 and send them out the door. I also gave them an informational sheet that explained the precautions to take with a head injury, like waking the patient every thirty minutes and making sure there were no severe headaches or vomiting, checking their pupils regularly for any signs of increased intracranial pressure. If any of those symptoms occurred, the patient would have to be seen again. I referred them to a specialist only if something was not normal.

I never had anyone bring a child back whom I had seen

with a head injury. I never missed one. Today in the US, if you have a kid with a head injury, a CT scan is automatically taken, even before the doctor sees the patient. That bill alone is about $6,000 to $7,000. On a typical night in the US, for only the single diagnosis of head injury in a child, several million dollars will be spent on CT scans and unnecessary exposure to radiation. And it costs you. It costs me. It costs all of us.

Of course, if there are symptoms of anything serious, tests must be ordered. My point is, as a physician gets older and more experienced, he or she can pick up on things. When a lady walks in, I can tell if she's got a problem or not. And 99% of the time I'm going to be right. Nowadays if you have pain in your lower right abdomen, a little fever, and nausea, they're automatically going to do a blood count and X-rays in order to rule out appendicitis. But if a doctor has seen patients hundreds of times with those symptoms, he or she will know when one or two of those situations might be appendicitis. For everyone else most of the time, the best advice is to go home for six or eight hours and come back if they're not feeling better. At least 99% of the time everything will be fine. But that doesn't happen anymore.

I took my very first vacation in the early 1980s. I went hunting with my uncle. A very good obstetrician was on call for me, and he gave my patient an epidural. There was a complication, and she couldn't breathe, had cardiac arrest, and died. Another obstetrician who was helping resuscitate her did an emergency C-section and delivered a healthy baby boy. I was devastated when I heard the news from my wife.

When I got back home, I drove sixty-five miles up to where the lady's family lived. They were very cold to me and blamed me for not being there for the delivery. Her father said I was a jokester because he had heard that I had a photo of Burt Reynolds on the ceiling of my exam room. He blamed me for everything, no matter what I said. I can understand that he was mad, because his daughter had died, which is something I fortunately have never experienced.

They ended up suing. They sued everybody: me, the doctor who gave the epidural, the emergency room doctor who tried to resuscitate the woman and was a cardiology fellow, the hospital, the doctor who did the C-section and saved the baby, and two drug companies because they didn't know which bupivacaine, Marcaine or Sensorcaine, had been used on her.

The attorney who took my deposition told me that I hadn't explained the epidural to the mother. But I had thoroughly documented notes covering everything. Then he asked if I had told her she could die from an epidural. I replied that I had explained everything to her about an epidural and had given her literature to read more about it, but I couldn't say definitely that I had said she could die from it. He then started insulting me, calling me all kinds of names, and telling me what a bad physician I was.

This went on for four years. After numerous depositions and postponed trails in an attempt to get me to settle, they decided to schedule a trial for the first week of December so they could march the little four-year-old boy in and say, right before Christmas, how sad it was that he didn't have a mother. The hospital had already settled. The doctor who did the epidural had filed for bankruptcy. Both drug companies had settled, and the emergency room doctor had settled. That left only the doctor who did the C-section and me.

The Sunday night before the trial was to begin, the doctor who did the C-section, his lawyer, and the plaintiff's lawyer went drinking together in a bar at the Holiday Inn in the town where the trial was to be held, and that doctor ended up settling. I have no doubt that the two lawyers split the money. That left only me.

My attorney called me late that night to tell me I had to settle. I said, "I'm not settling, because I didn't do anything wrong."

She said, "But you don't understand. Don't you know about joint and several liability?" She went on to explain that even if they found me only 2 or 3% liable, I could potentially be held accountable for the entire amount of the judgment. They wouldn't be telling the jury that all the others in the case had already settled because the suit was only against me. The jury would never know that the plaintiff had already received money from the hospital, from the other doctor, from the emergency room doctor, and from the two drug companies. That meant if they found me only a little bit liable—as little as 3 or 4%—the judgment could end up holding me 100% liable because it would be perceived that there was no one else to take up the slack in the money. I repeated, "I'm not going to settle."

The next morning someone from my insurance company showed up. He, too, told me to settle because if I didn't, I was going to be personally responsible for the amount of money above the amount my insurance company was willing to settle for. If the insurance company would settle for $600,000, for example, and I got a $4 million judgment against me, I would be responsible for $3.4 million.

"You've got to be kidding me!"

"No, he said. "That's the way it works."

"I'm going to trial!" I said.

Even my uncle called me, begging me to settle, which eventually I had to do, but it made me bitter as hell.

That was the beginning of eleven years of misery.

My second lawsuit involved a lady who had come to me with a one-week history of breast tenderness. This was right before her period was to start. I'd never seen her before. She was about thirty-six years old. When I checked her, she was tender on palpation and had some nodularity in her breast, which most women do. I told her to come back in three months. If anything got worse, she was to come back sooner. I also told her to cut back on coffee, tea, cokes, and chocolates. I dictated everything in her chart and noted that if things weren't better when she returned, we were going to do a mammogram. Two and a half years later she showed up again, without ever having come back to see me before then, and had an inflammatory carcinoma of the breast, which is a very aggressive tumor.

She died, and her husband sued me. His lawyer was a young guy about my age who was known for suing everybody. He had even been picked up for cocaine possession once but was let off the hook. When the lawyer deposed me, he told me not to take it personally, even though he was drawing out the process. He'd schedule a time for the deposition, and then he'd cancel it. We'd schedule another meeting, and I'd cancel all my office appointments. The day before the deposition was to take place, he'd call and say he was changing it to another day. Later, he scheduled the trial, and I cleared out a whole week of appointments. The Friday afternoon before the week of the trial, he cancelled and said they were postponing it for three months. He did that several times. He was trying to aggravate me so that I would settle, but I was not going to settle because I wasn't wrong.

His argument was that I should have called the lady

in three months' time and made her come in to see me again. I never do something like that. No one does! She was personally responsible.

Before the trial, they couldn't find anyone in the state of Texas who would come in as an expert witness against me. They ended up finding a doctor in Illinois, a hired gun whom they flew down to testify. He walked into the courtroom with a sport coat on and a damned stethoscope sticking out of his pocket. He testified that I was negligent.

My attorney asked him when was the last time he'd examined a lady with a breast problem. He answered, "Oh, about eight or ten years ago." Then how could he could be such an expert, my lawyer asked. The trial lasted all week, and on Friday afternoon it took the jury about five minutes to find me not guilty. Doctors see hundreds of women every day with premenstrual tenderness and nodularity in the breast. If they all ordered mammograms for their patients, thousands of women would be needlessly exposed to X-rays and costs would soar.

There was another case when I was covering for a doctor. A lady came in who was about seventeen weeks pregnant with twins. When I checked her, she was five to six centimeters dilated and her membranes were bulging. She, in effect, was having a late miscarriage. When I was in the next room delivering a term pregnancy, she started delivering the twins. As soon as I was done, I ran over to deliver the placenta. The twins were not viable. I did a thorough exam and dictated in detail that the placentas were of normal size, the blood loss was normal, and there were no lacerations.

I put her in a hospital room and went to see her the next day. Her blood count was normal so I sent her home so she wouldn't have to be in the ward with a bunch of women and their newborn babies—to get her out of there for emotional reasons. The last thing she needed was to hear crying babies or see women carrying their babies back and forth.

A few weeks after she delivered, she started complaining of bleeding and went to see her original doctor. He decided to do a D&C—dilation and curettage, a procedure to remove tissue from the inside of the uterus—because she was bleeding so much. While doing the D&C, he perforated her uterus. Then, of all things, he thought she needed a hysterectomy and did one right then.

He told her the reason for the D&C was because there was placenta still in the uterus. Then she sued me because she said I had left placenta in her uterus. When the pathologist looked at the scrapings from the D&C and the uterus after the hysterectomy, he found no evidence of placental tissue, and her blood count had been normal, which indicated that there was little blood loss.

There was no trial, but it went back and forth for nearly two years, after every doctor who looked at the evidence kept saying that I hadn't done anything wrong. But, of course, my insurance company had to get involved, and then my attorney. I had to deal with all that crap. I'd wake up in the middle of the night thinking about it, on top of the stress of doing surgeries and delivering babies.

I was furious. All those damn trial lawyers trying to win the lottery. They were just fishing for a case. They looked at doctors like we were the ticket. A lot of the trial lawyers, especially in Grayson County, were in bed with the judges. They were all as crooked as a barrel of snakes. Call an ace an ace and a spade a spade! If the shoe fits, wear it!

All any of this does is create anger. Doctors start practicing defensive medicine, and health care costs go up and up and up! Trust me, it is going to continue to go up if something isn't done about it. I will guarantee you that your insurance premiums are going up and this Obamacare is the biggest farce in the world. That's another book by itself.

There was another case. A lady came to see me because she wasn't getting pregnant. I did a laparoscopy—a procedure for looking into the abdomen by inserting a small tube in the umbilicus—and found out that she had endometriosis, which is extremely common. I treated her with medication for the endometriosis in hopes that she would get pregnant.

She moved to another town, which was about 200 miles away. At one point she called me from Arkansas and told me what had been going on with her. "Mary," I said, "you've got a tubal pregnancy." She wanted to come see me, but I told her that it was too far and too dangerous. She could bleed to death. I told her to go to the emergency room at Sparks Memorial Hospital in Fort Smith, which I knew because my family had used it. I told her to tell them that she'd spoken with me, that I'd done a laparoscopy, that she had endometriosis, and that I thought she had a pregnancy in her tube.

Sure enough, she did have a tubal pregnancy. The doctor treated her, and she went home. During the follow-up visit, he did a Pap smear, which came back normal.

Three or four months later she moved back to Oklahoma, close to the Texas border. She came to see me and said again that she wanted to get pregnant. So I put her back on the medicine to suppress the endometriosis and told her that there was an increased risk of another tubal pregnancy. When she had completed the course of the medication, she called me saying that she had missed a period. I told her that she needed to come in so I could see her. She wanted to come immediately, but I was headed to the hospital to deliver twins. I told her to come in the afternoon that same day at two.

That made her mad. She wanted to come in right then and there. So she ended up going to see a doctor located in a town a bit closer to where she lived. It took him about three to four weeks to diagnose that she had another pregnancy in her tube and decide to operate on her. Then he did a Pap smear, and it showed she had cancer of the cervix. He told her to sue me because I hadn't done a Pap smear when I saw her after she had moved back from Arkansas.

On my chart, I noted that I had sent for her records, that a Pap smear had been done in Fort Smith, and that it had been normal. I didn't do a new Pap smear because it had only been three months since the previous one. She was young and had never had an abnormal Pap smear. Her previous Pap smears were all normal, so why do one? If I had, it would have been seen as doing an extra Pap smear only to charge more money.

She sued me. Her uncle was a trial lawyer in Tulsa who at one time had run for governor of Oklahoma. He started calling and harassing me. I told him there was no way it was my fault. He'd call at night. He'd call me at the office. I told him to go to hell. I told him, "I'm tired of this crap. I didn't do anything wrong." This went on for two or three years. Once again, I called my insurance company, who now knew I had another lawsuit against me, and once again, I hired an attorney.

Finally, one afternoon her lawyer came to my office to get a deposition. My attorney drove up from Dallas to be there, too. I told them exactly what had happened. I told them the other doctor was jealous of me because I had such a big practice. Her uncle stood up and announced that there was nothing to sue me on. I wanted to punch him in the damned nose. He'd put me through hell for more than two years.

I got bitter. It made me want to do a Pap smear on every woman who walked in the door and practice more defensive medicine.

Another lawsuit involved a patient of my associate. She was pregnant and called in saying she was running a fever and thought she had a kidney infection. I told her to come in, but she didn't, and I made a note of that in her chart.

The next night, she went to the hospital and her doctor, my associate, was on call. He admitted her with a diagnosis of a severe kidney infection. She had had an argument with her husband and gone out walking in the streets in the rain and cold. Within twenty-four hours she was comatose.

The next night I went to see her in the hospital when I was on call. I'd never seen her before, and there was no change in her condition. She ended up dying, and the family sued all of us. Yet again, my insurance company was notified, and I had to get a lawyer. I had to do a deposition and go through the whole long, drawn-out process. After about three years, it went to trial. Eventually, they dropped the charges against me after I testified.

All this crap went on for eleven straight years. It's an unbelievable amount of stress. How could I go home at night, see my family, and be in a good mood knowing that others wanted to take me down? At the same time, I was trying to take good care of my patients and keep them from dying. Why would any person want to go through all that? My dad used to beg me to quit. He would say, "Son, you don't need to do this. It's going to kill you. Basta! Basta! Enough!" He saw a change in my personality. Of course, I wanted to greet everyone with a smile, but after a while I started looking at each patient as a possible litigant.

Those were extremely stressful years, and I became bitter because of the system, the lawyers, and the crooks. Suddenly, I found myself doing an extra Pap smear on a lady who didn't need it because I remembered the woman who had sued me. All any of this litigation does is drive up the cost of health care.

I also became less generous. Instead of not charging or reducing the cost of my services for patients like I used to do, I had to start charging everyone. Why? Because I had to pay for documentation and additional insurance. I had to spend one and a half to two hours every night dictating my charts for my transcriptionist to make sure I had everything covered. Today, when you go to see a doctor, it's all about the electronic medical records (which is another racket). The doctors and nurses are writing everything on the computer. When I took my mother to a doctor recently, he spent all of his time with his back to her, writing down her history. He hardly had time to exam her, he was so busy documenting everything because a lawyer would be looking at his charts. Do you blame him? He could not stand it but if you don't, look out! It's insane!

Medicine is all about big business now. Everyone is so greedy. Now there are degree programs in hospital administration. Administrators get paid $750,000, $1 million, dollars, even $2 million to run private hospitals, which is a lot more than doctors make. Administrators train a quarter of the time a doctor does and have a fraction of the stress to deal with. They have their own "fraternity."

All the Catholic hospitals, the Methodist and Baptist hospitals that were charity hospitals in the past have been bought out by private companies. It's what I call the upside down pyramid. The base of the pyramid used to be the health care providers and at the top was an administrator. Now the pyramid has been turned upside down and all the administrative people are at the top and the health care providers are the little part at the bottom. There are more administrative people now than people taking care of patients.

Health care used to constitute 8 to 10% of the GNP, the gross national product. Now it's 20%. The big private hospital chains are getting filthy rich. It's all about greed. They don't give a damn about the patient. They've created an environment in which people going into medicine now want to work eight hours a day, four days a week. They don't want to come in after hours. There are hospitalists now, who are doctors hired by the hospital to provide all care in the hospital. The hospitalist will take the patient's history and do the physical. The internist who may have taken care of a person for ten, fifteen, twenty, or thirty years may not even come in to see the person. Why? Because the hospital wants to charge for the services of the doctor they hired. That way they make more money. And the hospital probably will end up hiring the internist, too, put him on a salary, and set him up in an office building next to the hospital. Administrators have figured out who brings in the most revenue and promote those specialties over others.

Private practice doctors have become extinct. They're like dinosaurs. The patient is just a pawn now, just a number. Our health care system has been destroyed. Big business has driven a big wedge between the patient and the doctor, which is a private, even sacred, relationship. The days of medicine being a *calling* are coming to an end.

I realized that I needed to get out.

I'm not mad at the world. I'm frustrated. I'm frustrated because so many people are going into medicine today only for the almighty dollar. When I went into medicine, it was because I thought it was a calling. I wanted to help people. Now people are going into it for the wrong reason. There aren't many physicians who are dedicated anymore.

When I started practicing medicine the maternal mortality rate was 5.5 per 100,000 in the United States. Now it's more than 50 per 100,000. That's due to the increase of C-sections. With C-sections women can die from anesthetic death, pulmonary embolus, or infection.

Thousands of women have had unnecessary C-sections. The number one reason for doing a C-section is convenience, and the number two reason is fetal monitoring. Nurses in OB units now sit out in the nurses' station watching a monitor and the baby's heartbeat on the screen. They don't go into the room and put a hand on the mother's abdomen to make sure she's having good contractions. They sit on their butts and watch the fetal monitor. Heaven forbid there should be a glitch. If they see there's fetal distress, they call the doctor who ends up doing a C-section. Back in the early 1970s, when they started doing fetal monitoring, the C-section rate went from 5 to 25%. Now it's up to around 40%.

Another reason there are so many C-sections is because of lawsuits against obstetricians, claiming they caused cerebral palsy. Doctors are increasingly under pressure to do a C-section so the baby doesn't end up becoming hypoxic—not having enough oxygen—and getting brain damage. The lawsuits continue in spite of the fact that we now know that, even with the increase in C-sections over the last thirty to forty years, the incidence of cerebral palsy has changed zero. In fact, recent studies indicate that most cerebral palsy and other abnormalities of the brain occur between weeks twenty and twenty-eight, probably due to some type of viral infection or other events happening during this time of the pregnancy.

They even tried to do a C-section on my youngest

daughter. For ten days her obstetrician also wanted to induce her labor, for convenience only, but my daughter and I told her not to mess with nature. Fortunately, my daughter's membranes had ruptured the night before she was scheduled to go into the hospital. I tried to be the grandfather and not the doctor, but my daughter wanted me with her. While I was talking to her, I put my hand on her abdomen. She was having piddly contractions. Next thing I knew, they had given her an epidural, which generally slows labor if it's given too early because of the numbing. Time went by, and she was still only two to three centimeters dilated. I went in a few more times to feel her tummy, and there was still no good pattern of labor. Nothing was happening. Then her doctor came in and said that if her labor didn't advance in the next hour or two, they were going to do a C-section.

I blew up. I walked in there and told the nurse, "Let me tell you, I'm an obstetrician. I've delivered more babies than you've probably ever even seen. I want you to do what I say and tell the doctor. I want the epidural turned off. I want her turned on her left side, and I want you to turn up the Pitocin"—the medicine that causes her contractions to increase. "I mean it," I said. Within an hour she was completely dilated. She pushed once, and the baby came out. Now that baby is seven years old and is my brilliant granddaughter.

I quit delivering babies on May 29, 1994. The stress

was too much. I decided to do only gynecology.

To the youngsters going into medicine, you better *not* go into it if you are going for the money. I tell you it is a *calling*. If you do, you take care of the *whole* patient. Do not compartmentalize your patient. Take a good history, look at and listen to them, put your hands on them and *not* the computer.

In my specialty, do a complete exam including a rectal. I cannot tell you how many rectal cancer and ovarian cancers I picked up by the rectal exam. If your OB-GYN does not do a rectal you better consider changing doctors. I found a carcinoma of the rectum on my twenty-eight-year-old patient, who later brought me a plaque showing the rear end of a car that stated, "Rear end checkups are priceless." Her life was saved by that rectal exam.

While I'm on the subject of history and physicals, instead of focusing on the patient and how to improve our diagnosis and treatment of the patient, our medical establishment is now spending all of our continuing medical education with a good portion of the courses and training on medical litigation: "How to avoid lawsuits," If it's not in this one, there are numerous courses on how your office needs to code your visit or surgery so they can maximize their reimbursement for the insurance company. Now, you tell me it is not all about the money!

I'm so proud to say when I was in medical school and residency we never, ever had a course on this because at that time, it was about taking care of the patient!

I know I'm not perfect, but a lot of people expect perfection. None of us is perfect. We all make mistakes.

My psychiatric professor in medical school used to tell us that it was going to be devastating when we lost a patient. He said, "If you practice medicine long enough and have done enough cases, you're going to lose a patient. It's going to happen to you. You better try to be prepared."

I lost three patients. One was a lady I had done a hysterectomy on for severe prolapse of the uterus. She was elderly, but she was doing great. I kept her in the hospital a little longer than usual because of her age. She was getting ready to go home, had her clothes on and everything, when she had a heart attack. It was totally unrelated to the surgery.

Then there was the lady that I had done a repeat C-section on. I offered her a VBAC, which means a vaginal birth after cesarean, but she didn't want it. She wanted another C-section, even though I told her the risk was higher. About twenty-four hours after the surgery, at around 4:30 a.m., she had a pulmonary embolus, a blood clot in her lung, and died. There was nothing I could have done for her. It was not my fault. I went to the autopsy, which was very traumatic for me, because I wanted to know the cause of her death. The C-section had been perfect, though there was a large clot in her lung. Later, I found out that a genetic predisposition for blood clots, known as the Factor V Leiden, had been discovered. She had two or three other close family members who had had a pulmonary embolus, so I suspect she, too, had the Factor V Leiden.

The third patient I lost was a lady I had done a laparoscopy on as an outpatient. She was obese, and a clamp came off during the procedure. I think when that happened, the needle I'd put through her belly button punctured a blood vessel. Eventually, she went into disseminated intravascular coagulopathy, or DIC. In other words, she had consumed all her clotting factors and couldn't clot anymore. She ended up brain dead and was taken off the respirator after two days, on October 25, 1998.

She was the only patient I ever lost like that, and it devastated me. The following Monday I forced myself to go back into the operating room to do the five cases I had scheduled. It was not easy to keep going, even knowing I was scheduled to retire in three weeks. I couldn't get the patient's family off my mind, and I thought of all the things they must be going through. Though I was severely depressed, I knew I couldn't give up. I had to keep going. It reminds me of the quote of Winston Churchill: "If you're going through hell just keep on going!"

One Saturday morning while I was in the bathtub, feeling sorrowful, I remembered what my high school football coach, Stan Funderburg, used to say. "One reason we play football," he said, "is to learn that later in life, when we get knocked on our rear, we have to pick ourselves up." I jumped out of the tub and told myself that I had to get on with my life. I had to make something positive out of this tragedy instead of wasting my time feeling sorry for myself.

I retired November 15, 1999, a year later than I had originally planned.

The story I want to tell is not about poor, pitiful me. I survived, and as a result, I was a stronger person and more determined than ever to make a difference in this world.

PART III

Giving Back

The Greatest Need

"If you don't stand for something, you'll fall for anything."

When I was a kid, missionaries would come to our church. A lot of them had worked in Africa and talked about how they ministered to people there. I was intrigued and very inquisitive about what went on. At the time, in the 1950s, there weren't digital cameras like we have now that can take lots of photos. They'd show maybe only one or two pictures, and I thought, "I want to see more! I want to go to Africa!"

So after I retired, the first thing I did was call the American College of Obstetrics and Gynecology. I told them that I wanted to do volunteer work and go to Africa, and asked if they knew of anywhere I could go. The woman I spoke with didn't know of anything, so I thought I'd call back in three or four weeks and try again, which I did. Same thing. They didn't have any avenues for people who wanted to donate their time, which I found very frustrating.

Later, when I was at a medical meeting in Dallas, I met a gentleman, a doctor, who knew something about doing missionary work. He gave me the name of a doctor to call. I called that doctor, and he asked me where I wanted to go. I said Africa. He said, "I can get you into Ghana."

I flew to Ghana by myself and landed late one night in Accra. I was the only white person I could see for miles. The person picking me up was two hours late, and it was hot, stuffy, and humid. I wondered what I'd gotten myself into.

We traveled for about five hours up through central Ghana to a village, Ankaase, where I stayed for three weeks, doing general practice work. It was very primitive. The people were so poor. Everyone was sick—the kids and the women and men, too. There were so many diseases: malaria, typhoid, pneumonia, rabies, tetanus. The kids would get tetanus of the umbilical cord when they were delivered because of the unclean environment. It was mind boggling to see the depths of poverty these people were living in.

I saw patients in a small clinic run by a Methodist mission. One case in particular was a real eye opener. A little girl had been bitten by a dog. If a dog is not vaccinated for rabies, it has to be isolated for two weeks. Of course, most of the dogs there were not vaccinated. I told the girl's family that they needed to isolate the dog and to come back and tell me what was going on.

Two or three days later they walked back and told me that the dog had been killed. I had told them not to kill the dog, but by the time they'd gotten back home, it was already dead. Then I asked them to bring the dog in so that we could send the brain off to be evaluated for rabies. They said, "Oh, we ate the dog."

• • •

It was so very hot in the village, and we were in the middle of what's called the harmattan. That's when Saharan winds from the northeast bring in sand and dust. I'd wake up in the middle of the night and could hardly breathe. Plus during that time of year, they do a lot of burning of the underbrush in order to be able to harvest during the rainy season and to catch animals. As the animals try to escape the fire, people capture and kill them to eat. I had to go outside all the time to be able to breathe.

A pregnant lady came in to give birth. While delivering her baby, she tore into the rectum. We didn't have any anesthesia or many instruments, and those we did have weren't much good. The needles were all the wrong size. While I was sewing her up, I stuck myself pretty badly. I was worried about HIV, which was prevalent at the time. We ran a test on her and, of all things, it came back positive.

I thought, "Oh my God. This is something. Here I am, my first trip to Africa, and I've stuck myself with a needle that may be infected with HIV." I called some doctors back in the US who I knew were dealing with infectious disease, and they told me what to do. I went to the city, bought two of the three medicines they recommended that were available, and started taking them. About five or six days later, we repeated the test on the lady for confirmation, and it came back negative. I was very fortunate!

I made three more trips back to Ghana that year. One was with an obstetrician/gynecologist who was doing maternal mortality studies and treatment. He had a foundation that was involved with the Catholic Church and the Vatican. I went around Ghana with him for three weeks.

I soon turned off because it didn't seem like he cared about his patients. He was cold as ice to them, but he was warm as sunshine to the administrative people he was dealing with. To me, he didn't have a very caring attitude. Sitting next to him in the airport on the way home, I asked to see the foundation's financials. Turns out he was getting a nice, cushy salary in excess of $100,000. His son, who wasn't a doctor, was also working for him and had a salary of around $60,000. And they were getting all their expenses paid for. I looked him straight in the eye and said, "I don't agree with this. If you're going to give, then give. I'm not going to take. I'm going to do something else." I parted ways with him.

The only good thing about being with that doctor was I met other people through him. I went to Ghana twice more that year, and four times within the next year and a half.

On my third and fourth trips, I went to a Baptist mission way up north in the country, almost to the border with Burkina Faso. It took about twelve hours to drive there from Accra. The village was very small and isolated. The doctor with whom I worked, Dr. George Faile, had been living there with his family for about twenty years. His father had started the clinic in 1957. There were three or four other doctors there, too. It was extremely impressive. They were so well organized. They were seeing 50,000 to 60,000 patients a year and doing around 1,500 surgeries. I was so impressed. They were so dedicated; they genuinely cared; and they did a lot of good work.

My son and a young female obstetrician/gynecologist went with me on my fourth trip. We had been up all night driving and were exhausted. I had drunk a lot of caffeine and eaten Hershey bars, and we were all dehydrated.

We arrived late at night and went around the ward. I couldn't believe my eyes. Five children in the pediatric ward had died that day from malaria. I couldn't wait to start helping.

The next day I did a C-section on a lady and resuscitated her baby. Everything went fine. Another pregnant lady was very sick. She was very lethargic and extremely anemic. Her blood count was so low that she needed a blood transfusion. My son, who was around eighteen at the time, and I both donated blood for her, but she died about twenty-four hours later. The next night at about 2:00 a.m., I woke up and my heart was beating very rapidly. It felt like it was 200 beats a minute. It scared me. I had never had anything like that happen before. There was no EKG machine available, and nothing they gave me would help. I was so weak, I had to leave. We traveled for eight hours and spent the night. After another six hours or so, I got on a plane and flew home. The cardiologist I saw once I was back in Texas said my blood pressure was high, and he put me on medication. I was determined to get back in shape and return to Africa.

I was doing mostly general medicine in Africa, but I what I really wanted to do was fistula treatment. I had met a doctor when I was doing my residency at Charity Hospital in New Orleans who had gone to Africa to work on obstetric fistulas. His name was Jack Robertson. He was twenty-five years my senior and a true gentleman with his white wavy hair, deep voice, and fine suit and bow tie.

Dr. Robertson had trained at the Tulane Service of Charity Hospital in the 1950s. He also had the distinction of being the father of urogynecology and, along with Karl

Storz, developed the first cystoscope for gynecological use. We chatted, and he told me about his time in Africa and the fistula work he'd done there. It really intrigued me, and I said to myself that when I could, that was what I wanted to do one day.

I hadn't heard of obstetric fistula before because it didn't exist in the United States. Fistula, by definition, is an abnormal communication between two organs. An obstetric fistula is a hole that is caused by an obstetrical event. It happens in women who are in labor for a very long time, and they can't deliver the baby for one of three reasons, often referred to as the "three Ps." The "Power" of the uterus pushes the "Passenger" (the baby) through the "Passageway" (the birth canal). If the passenger is too large for the passageway, or if the passageway is too small for the passenger, or if the power of the uterus cannot push the passenger through the passageway, there is a problem and a C-section is necessary, ideally, within 24 hours of the onset of labor.

Due to the lack of health care facilities and adequate health care workers in Third World countries, the process of giving birth under these difficult circumstance can go on for days, or even weeks, as inconceivable as that seems. It is one of the contributing factors to the extremely high maternal and infant mortality rates in those countries. When I first started going to Sierra Leone, the maternal and infant mortality rate there was the highest in the world, according to the United Nations. Even today in Sierra Leone, a woman has a one-in-eight chance of dying from childbirth during her lifetime, and one of three children under the age of five dies from disease.

There are three obstacles in the Third World to women having early access to C-sections. The first is the traditional birth attendant, or TBA. A TBA is a woman in the village who has no formal training in delivering babies. She may keep a birthing woman in the village too long for financial reasons. Of the first 500 women we saw, the average length of labor was four to five days. That is mind boggling! I treated two women who had been in labor for fifteen days and survived!

The second obstacle is getting to a facility quickly enough. It may take days to walk out of the bush and through rivers and creeks to reach a facility. Sometimes the birthing mother is carried in a hammock or on a motorbike. The third obstacle is the lack of money to pay for the C-section once the mother arrives at a facility, assuming the facility has the capacity to do a C-section in the first place, which is not often the case.

It's sad to say that if the mother doesn't die from infection, hemorrhage, or a ruptured uterus, 98% of the time the unborn baby will die. Depending on how the baby is positioned in the mother's uterus, the presenting part, which is generally the head, gets stuck in the pelvis. The constant pressure cuts off the blood supply to tissues in the vagina and bladder that lie between the head and pubic bone, and to the tissues in the vagina and rectum that lie between the head and the tailbone. If enough tissue dies between the head and the pubic bone, a hole, i.e., fistula, will develop between the bladder and vagina. This is called a vesico-vaginal fistula (VVF). About 4% of the time with a VVF, the tissue between the head and the tailbone will die also and a hole between the rectum and vagina develops. This is called a recto-vaginal fistula (RVF); it's also known as an obstetric fistula, which is a fistula as the result of an obstetrical event. It causes women to have an uncontrollable loss of urine and/or feces that runs down their legs.

Obstetric fistula has existed since the beginning of humankind. It has even been found in mummies of Egyptian queens. Until the twentieth century, every country in the world had women with obstetric fistulas. Now they exist only in women in Third World countries, thanks to modern obstetrics, which makes it possible to deliver a baby with forceps or via a C-section within a reasonable twenty-four to thirty-six hours.

The first hospital to treat obstetric fistula in the United States was founded in New York City in 1855. J. Marion Sims was the first doctor to repair a vesico-vaginal fistula.

It's possible for a fistula to heal on its own if it's small enough and if a catheter is immediately inserted in the bladder to drain the urine. But in Africa today, women with long labors aren't seen soon enough. A woman with a fistula may not be seen for four or five years. I saw one woman who was sixty-seven years old, and she had had a fistula since she was a teenager. Urine had been pouring uncontrollably down her legs for fifty-one years.

Until recently, almost all women in Africa with a fistula were shunned by their villages. They were made fun of and ostracized because they smelled. Other women would have nothing to do with them. Sometimes they were tied to a tree and left to die. I read that four or five women chained themselves together, jumped into a river, and committed suicide.

After my last trip to Ghana, I received an email from a Peace Corps volunteer named Tom Johnson who had worked in Sierra Leone in the 1990s. He had heard that I wanted to work on fistulas and told me that I should go to Sierra Leone. He said there was a great need for doctors to do fistula surgery there. He told me to get in touch with a woman named Mimi Gettinger, who goes to Sierra Leone regularly to take care of amputees from the civil war. He also recommended that I speak with a plastic surgeon, Dr. Ian Zlotolow. He told me the same thing—that Mimi Gettinger would get me where I needed to be.

I got in to touch with Mimi and told her that I wanted to go to Sierra Leone to do fistula surgery. She said, "Okay, meet me in London, and I'll take you there."

We flew into Lungi Airport near Freetown, the capital and largest city of Sierra Leone, in November 2002. Then we got on a huge, old Sikorsky helicopter piloted by a bunch of Russian mercenaries and flew across the bay to the city. This was always a dicey experience as the Russians were known for overloading the helicopter with passengers and luggage, which led to several crashes. Once an entire soccer team perished in a helicopter crash. The other options were to drive more than three hours around the bay, take a ferry as slow as homemade molasses, board a small dangerous boat, or take the hovercraft that caught fire once in the middle of the bay. The tide once grounded the ferry in the middle of the bay and stranded one of our volunteers, Helen Weld, all night, sitting around waiting on the tide to come back up. It was a toss-up every time we had to decide which ride to take.

At the time, there were 17,500 UN troops in Sierra Leone. We stayed in a hotel where a lot of the UN people were staying. Mimi, who is very dramatic and overbearing, went up to some of the UN people and told them that she had a doctor from the United States with her whom she wanted to show around the country. "I'm taking care of amputees," she said, "and I want a vehicle." Lo and behold, the UN gave her a vehicle with a driver, and for three weeks we went around Sierra Leone.

Driving through Freetown was like being in a war zone. Many buildings and infrastructure in this once-peaceful town were destroyed. It reminded me of my home town after the May 5, 1960 tornado. One of the first places we stopped was Connaught Hospital. It was a huge old dilapidated hospital that was like a ghost town. It was bare. Nothing was going on there, so we went to Princess Christian Maternity Hospital, sometimes referred to as The Cottage.

We walked in and discovered that it was primarily a hospital for obstetrics and gynecology. On Ward Five, there was a program for obstetric fistula that had been started that July by International Medical Corps. I thought I'd died and gone to heaven. There was a slew of patients with fistula. The doctor wasn't there, but I met with some of the nurses, who were very nice, and I thought, "This is what I want to do!"

I went back to Princess Christian the next day, and the doctor, who was Egyptian, was there. He was very nice to me, and I watched a few surgeries. But he had a temper and threw his instruments and screamed and yelled. Even though he treated me well, I knew that it could be difficult to work there.

Next we went up-country to Bo, the second largest city in Sierra Leone. The largest hospital in the country is located there and has many small wards for twenty to forty patients.

The Bo hospital was dilapidated, too, and it had a fence around it. There was no water and no electricity. The head of the hospital was Dr. Tom Rogers. He was a general practitioner and a surgeon, and he did everything.

They had an amputee ward, an infant-feeding ward full of malnourished kids, a pediatric ward, a general medicine ward, a general surgery ward, an obstetric ward, and a gynecology ward. They had occupancy for up to 400 people, but there were only 100 to 200 people there at the time. The hospital had all this capacity but rarely had electricity, and water had to be hand-carried from a well. It's amazing how the doctors there do what they do with so little. They have to improvise so much. I have very fond memories of Dr. Rogers, because he was always very kind to me. He succumbed to Ebola in 2014.

The hospital was very poorly furnished. They were short of sutures. They were short of IV fluids. They were short of everything. They simply had to make do. They didn't have a choice. They had to operate in the dark. I felt so sorry for them. A lot of people died because they didn't have the supplies they needed. I was there five days and couldn't get over what I was seeing. I'd never seen anything like it in my life.

I said to myself, "Oh my God. I've got to come back here."

Then we went back to Freetown, and I spent another five days with the doctor and nurses at Princess Christian Maternity Hospital. I got to know the nurses well and the two female Sierra Leonean doctors who were there, Dr. Virginia George and Dr. Alyona Lewis. They were understudies who were helping the Egyptian doctor.

When I left the country, I told them that I would call on a regular basis to see how things were going. In February or March 2003 I called, and they told me that the Egyptian doctor was leaving in May, and they were going to shut down the program. I said, "Okay, I'm coming over. Keep all the equipment. Keep everything going, and I'll come."

I went back to Freetown and met with the head of Princess Christian hospital. I told him that I would come on a regular basis and bring money to feed the patients if he would let me operate in the hospital. Dr. Lewis and Dr. George would help me. Dr. Lewis had surgical experience doing fistulas and was good at it, but she hadn't had access to gynecological training. She and I would do simple surgeries. Then when I'd go back home, I could send money, and she could do a few surgeries. So I started going back and forth three times a year, staying in Sierra Leone for two or three weeks at a time doing surgeries.

After my third trip in 2004, I realized we needed to be a foundation so I started the West Africa Fistula Foundation. I created a 501(c)(3) in the United States and an NGO, a non-governmental organization, in Africa. Mimi Gettinger had introduced me to the wife of a gentleman who ran her organization. We spent two solid weeks in Sierra Leone going from one office to another, doing all the administrative work, which was a big pain and, in the end, it was all about money. Everywhere we went, we had to pay: $1,000 here, $500 there, $700 somewhere else.

I used all of my own money, and it wore me out. At that time, we had used vehicles that were not in good shape. On several occasions when there were fuel shortages, we had to pay through the nose for black market fuel. I can't remember how many times we ran out of fuel because our gauges were not working, and we were stranded for hours. I ran out of toes and fingers counting the number of times we had punctures (flat tires).

For about another year, until the middle of 2005, I continued to do surgeries at the Princess Christian Maternity Hospital. The conditions, however, were deplorable. I had to pay for diesel to turn the generator on, and half the time it wouldn't work. But we kept seeing patients and doing surgeries. Benjamin Rogers, Dr. Rogers' nephew, would work out of Bo and bring us sometimes twenty-five patients on the bus for us to operate on in Freetown.

Theresa Tkacik, who also happened to be from Texas, worked as a nurse practitioner at the US Embassy in Freetown. She had heard about us and would often come to the hospital. She loved what we were doing. One day I told her that I needed to leave Princess Christian because the conditions were so bad. I needed to find somewhere else to do surgeries. She told me about a place on Signal Hill called Choithram Hospital. It had been a British colonial hospital, and the Jordanians, who ran it during the war, were getting ready to move out in December. I decided to try to move up there.

Choithram was a much better facility than Princess Christian. It had twenty-four-hour electricity and water, and two well-lit operating rooms. I spent weeks finding out who was on the hospital's board. Initially, they were hesitant to have us rent the facility because of the stigma of fistula, even though the hospital was nearly empty. I ended up offering them $3,500 a month for use of the facility. For that, they would give me two wards for four patients each and access to the operating room almost any time I wanted it.

I kept our patients down at Princess Christian Maternity Hospital until we were ready to operate on them. Then we'd take eight patients at a time up to Choithram, operate on them, and keep them there for three or four days. When they were doing okay, I'd send them back to Princess Christian and have eight others sent up.

The first year at Choithram we did 215 surgeries. The second year we did 221. The third year, all of a sudden, after four months, we had done only 39 surgeries. I found out that people were "eating the money." In other words, there was corruption, which is something I cannot stand. I immediately put a halt to it and realized it was time to move on.

That's when I decided to leave Freetown and go up-country to Bo, where the fistulas really were.

The majority of the fistulas I see in Africa are very large and require a complex operation to repair them. About 10 to 15% are so bad they are irreparable and can't be operated on. In those cases, we do a urinary diversion, which entails making a bladder from the intestines and diverting to outside of the abdomen. We use a continence mechanism, which eliminates the need to wear an appliance or bag. Though this remains a controversial procedure, many patients would rather risk the procedure than live with their condition.

Because fistulas don't occur anymore in the West, physicians don't learn how to do the surgery to repair them in their residency program. Many doctors go to Africa without a clue as to how to fix a fistula, and sometimes they end up making things worse. The unfortunate thing is that the first chance for repairing a fistula is usually the best chance there is.

I learned to do fistula repair surgery by starting on small, simple fistulas and gradually doing more difficult ones. I was more or less self-taught, but I already had a lot of experience doing vaginal surgeries, so I was comfortable with the anatomy. But the whole thing was unlike anything I'd ever seen before. Often when I bring very experienced people to Sierra Leone and show them fistulas for the first time, they can't believe what they're seeing. They will say that they don't know how I do it. I tell them it takes experience.

When I went up to Bo, I found out about Holy Mary, an old Catholic hospital that had been built by a Sierra

Leonean doctor. He had gone to Italy for his training and married an Italian pediatrician who was Catholic. They had been able to get money through the Vatican to build the hospital in Bo.

The doctor also started a nursing school next to the hospital. Unlike his wife, he was self-serving. He charged the nurses for their training even though the school wasn't accredited. Students thought they were going to come out with a degree, but they didn't. The guy was only after their money. He also got involved politically and at one time ran for president.

He came to Freetown, where he had a practice, and left the hospital in Bo empty. I met with him, and we made a deal that I would pay half of the expenses if he'd let me move in. At the time, it was a halfway decent hospital. We agreed that we'd figure out the expenses once I got there. Right before I was to get on the airplane to fly up to Bo, he sent an email saying that he wanted $22,000 for me to move in. I said no way, I wasn't going to do it. Then he tried to keep me from getting out all our equipment and supplies that we had already moved into the hospital.

By the time this was going on, Dr. Koroma was already working at the government hospital in Bo. Through a Sierra Leonean friend of mine, Samuel Pieh, who knew the minister of health, I had been able to get Dr. Koroma, who was the only OB-GYN in the entire country outside of Freetown, transferred from Kenema to Bo. I did this because I needed to have a doctor in Bo who could do follow-ups on the surgeries I'd be doing and to care for my patients when I wasn't there. When Dr. Koroma heard about what was happening with Holy Mary Hospital, he said that I should forget about it and come to the Bo Government Hospital. He said he'd give me a ward. My Sierra Leonean staff got all our things out of Holy Mary in less than eight hours, and we moved into the government hospital.

We stayed at the Bo Government Hospital for seven years, until July 2015. We could handle as many as fifty patients at a time on the ward. For the first four years, there was no running water and no electricity 70% of the time. The generator didn't work, so to have any electricity at all, we had to rely on a water-powered plant that worked only during the wet season. We had to pay a lot of money for diesel when the generator, which was large and inefficient, was working to be able to do surgeries.

I went to Bo at least three times a year, generally for about three weeks at a time. I'd do all the fistula surgeries, usually within ten days, and then I'd spend another ten days making sure the patients were doing okay. I also did any other surgeries that were needed, like C-sections and hysterectomies. I even operated on kids with typhoid fever. I will never forget the man who carried his six-year-old daughter with her tummy so swollen and begged for help. It was obvious she needed surgery and I took her to the operating room. She had a bowel perforation as a consequence of advanced typhoid. Though I'm not a pediatric surgeon, I did what I had to do so she wouldn't die. How gratifying it was to see her up and running around a few days later!

I also treated a lot of women who came in in shock, having had a criminal abortion. Obviously, people didn't know what they were doing. Many women suffered from a perforated bowel and other complications due to these illegal procedures.

Then I'd go back to the US, and the nurses and Dr. Koroma would take care of the patients postoperatively, send the patients home, and bring in another group of patients. We fed the women and got them nourished. We found that it was extremely important that the women were well fed and nourished before we operated on them because of the parasitic diseases, such as malaria, they had. Also, they were often very anemic. We had to build up their systems in order for them to be able to tolerate the surgery.

After a while I hired Dr. Augustine Mannah, a general surgeon. He is almost my age and had served in the Sierra Leonean Army, where he had extensive experience taking care of war victims. When he got out of the army, he started working for NGOs. He was not a government employee like most doctors in Sierra Leone. Dr. Mannah continues to work with me now and is starting to do the simple cases like I did when I first started. He is a tremendous asset to our program as he takes care of the patients after I leave and does free C-sections on the patients we have repaired who get pregnant. We discourage them from delivering vaginally, because they are more than likely going to develop another fistula.

• • •

When I went back home to Texas, people started finding out about what I was doing in Sierra Leone, and I began doing some fundraising for the West Africa Fistula Foundation. Years ago, I had a patient who had delivered a stillborn baby early in her pregnancy. I had come in on my weekend off to take care of Elsie Stumpff and spent the night at the hospital with her and her husband, Kurt. Then she got pregnant again and had a little girl, whom I delivered. For some reason, they thought I had done something special. In appreciation, they wrote a check to the Foundation for over $300,000. They have continued to support the Foundation and are one of our main donors, giving a total of nearly a million dollars. They are common, hard-working, honest, frugal, conservative people who have a passion for helping others. They're one of our main donors.

Other major donors include the country singer Reba McEntire, who was my patient for years and has given hundreds of thousands of dollars, and Charlie Evans, from Colleyville, Texas, managing partner of Vandergriff Toyota in Arlington, Texas, who has generously helped with paying rent and renovating our new facility. Then there are the two amazing young ladies, Maria and Julia Myers, who created a non-profit, prettypurposeful.org. They have raised over $100,000 for us and continue to help the Foundation.

I started sending out newsletters and giving talks. Occasionally, someone sends $5, $50, or a $100. A minister whose wife I operated on years ago sends us $250 on a regular basis. It really touches me how people give. An older lady, bless her heart, used to send me $10. She called me one time and said she had landed on hard times and couldn't give anymore. I said to her, "My God, you've done great. That $10 a year meant so much to me." I told her what $10 could do in Africa, and how wonderful she was. I meant every word.

Every penny that's donated goes to Sierra Leone. We have zero administrative costs in the US. Zero. There's probably no other nonprofit in the United States that can say that.

To make a living after I retired, I started doing real estate along with my son Deno. (Wonder where he got that name?) We have continued the Maggi and Son logo, and in 2021, we will celebrate 100 years. I have an office in Denison, Texas, and I hired a woman named Jimi Lou Coleman to help me with the business and with the Foundation. I personally pay her salary. I pay for printing the newsletter and the postage. I pay my airfare to Africa. I do this so the Foundation will be squeaky clean.

If the Foundation spends roughly $180,000 to $200,000 a year, which doesn't include the money I spend, and we do 180 surgeries a year, it costs us $1,000 per surgery. It includes nurses' salaries, food (we feed the patients three meals a day), transportation (we send vehicles all over the country and out into the bush to bring patients to us because no one can afford to drive), fuel, medicine, IVs, taxes in Sierra Leone, NGO fees, everything. It's a bargain. A similar surgery in the US would easily cost $40,000 or more. It's hard to believe, but we, being an NGO, have to pay the Sierra Leonean government to work in the country. It can be as high as US$2,000 per year. We also have to pay withholding taxes, etc.

The West Africa Fistula Foundation doesn't receive financial support from agencies, such as USAID (United States Agency for International Development) or UNFDA (United Nations Population Fund), which establish quotas and other constraints. The Foundation has never received any public money. It's all privately funded.

At one time the British government had given more than £20 million to Sierra Leone to cover free health care services for women, pregnant women, and children under five. I'm sure that, at most, only one-fourth of that money ever got to the patients. People stole the money. People in Sierra Leone ate it. It's a terrible situation. There is still so much corruption in the country.

People ask me why I keep doing this, and I tell them that what keeps me going is the patients. It's my calling.

• • •

March 2014 was my last trip to Sierra Leone before the Ebola outbreak reached Bo. When I left, Ebola was already in eastern Sierra Leone, about seventy miles away. Six weeks later, people started dying by the hundreds.

A week after I got home, I became very sick and was hospitalized for eleven days. I ran a very high fever, couldn't eat for ten days, and lost twenty-five pounds. No one knew what was wrong with me. I was sick as a dog and thought I was going to die. I even named my pallbearers. I was weak for two months.

We ran Ebola tests about six months later, as well as a test for Lassa fever, which is endemic to the region. It's a virus similar to Ebola but not as bad, although it's highly contagious. I tested negative for both.

Because of the Ebola epidemic, the government had asked to take over our ward at the Bo Government Hospital. A volunteer, Paul Robinson, started working with us in 2010 when his extremely talented wife, Andrea, a nurse with midwifery and tons of administrative experience, came to Sierra Leone with Volunteer Services Overseas. Andrea was helping out at the Bo Government Hospital.

She and Paul liked what they saw with our organization. Paul eventually went to work with us. There is not one thing he can't do with the exception of one thing—birth a baby. Besides his incredible talent, he has tremendous compassion for the patients. Before he even started to work with us, he would come and tell us to take care of this patient and that patient, and he'd pay for it. Paul went back to Sierra Leone right after the Ebola crisis had ended. He called and told me that we were not going to be able to go back to our ward at the government hospital.

Fortunately, six months previously, Dr. Mannah had come across an old WHO (World Health Organization) HIV facility. It was a thirty-four-bed facility located in a valley on five acres of land that no one had been using because of the stigma of HIV. It sat there empty so we leased it for our excess patients.

Paul decided he was going to build an operating room at the facility. He came to the US and spent three weeks figuring out how to put one together. He told me that he wanted to get the facility ready for doing surgeries. He was going to install two generators so we would have twenty-four-hour electricity. He was going to put in a pump for twenty-four-hour water. And he was going to put an air conditioner in the operating room. All those years I'd been going to Africa, I never had an air conditioner, except at Choithram. When I did surgeries, my scrubs would be soaked, and I would have to wring them out.

On my next trip back to Bo, in August 2015, I arrived at a fully equipped facility that can accommodate up to forty-five patients. I named it Paul's Valley. In addition to the new surgical suite, it now has a beautiful, independent kitchen with storeroom, a generator room with ample space for a workshop and fuel storage, and remodeled showers and toilets, though many of the patients still prefer to sneak out to the bush instead.

Now that we have our own facility, we need $25,000 a month to keep things running. I'm the world's worst at asking for money. My wife gets aggravated with me because she says I'm not asking for myself.

What I want is a capital campaign. I want to raise $5 to $10 million so that with the interest, we won't need to worry about raising money anymore.

The need is so great in Sierra Leone. Because of the civil war, hospitals were destroyed everywhere, and doctors fled the country. Before the war, there were probably 500 to 600 doctors in Sierra Leone. After, there were maybe fifty or sixty total to serve a country about the size of South Carolina and with a population of around six million. And it's gotten even worse since the Ebola epidemic. There's an enormous need for health care facilities, and for water and electricity. The majority of facilities still don't have either. Today in Bo, which is the country's second largest city, electricity is available only about 35% of the time. Nurses often work without getting paid. For months, they go to work every day, because they hope one day they'll get paid.

It's an entirely different world. In the Bo Government Hospital today, the situation is just as bad as it was when I first went there in 2002. The poverty and corruption are incomprehensible. Human life has very little value. Once we had a lady who needed blood. We asked her husband to donate, and he said, "No. If she dies, I'll just get myself a new wife."

There are several things that keep me going. One is I can still do a lot of good in Sierra Leone and, hopefully, at some point in my lifetime before I die, we'll be able to change things. We're trying. The other thing is that we can do so much with so little.

There is nothing more meaningful or more gratifying for me than the work I do in Sierra Leone. I love it. The only reason I don't stay there is because I'm married and have a family in Texas.

My Patients' Stories

"Success breeds success."

Patients came in on stretchers. They came in wheelchairs. Some women were on crutches, because they literally could not ambulate. Yatta was skin and bones when she came to see us. She was literally just some skin wrapped around a bunch of bones. She couldn't even stand up to be weighed. The nurse had to help her stand on the scales. She didn't weigh more than seventy pounds. She was so weak and so malnourished. To see a lady like that—so poor, so distraught, so ostracized—and after two to three months of a regular diet, iron, vitamins, nutritional support, mental support, psychological support, she walks out of the hospital a new person is so gratifying. Nothing in this world could make me feel any better. You could give me $10 million, and it wouldn't come close to the amount of gratification and pleasure it gives me to see the change in these women's lives.

When I saw Memuna in 2003, she was irreparable. Everywhere she went, people told her that they couldn't do anything for her. She had a very bad fistula, her vagina was completely shut, and was spilling urine and feces. When she was fourteen, her father had sold her off to be married, and not long after, she had a labor that lasted for seven days.

Memuna didn't want to leave us once she had come to the hospital. She would do anything as long as she could stay. The nurses were willing to keep her, and she started working as a cleaner. Every day she went upstairs three times a day to pray that someone would help her. I told her that one day I was going to bring in a specialist to do her surgery. I didn't have the expertise or the facilities and equipment to do it.

After a couple of years, I brought a urological oncologist to Bo, and he did a urinary diversion on Memuna. It worked beautifully. Then we hired Memuna and eventually sent her to a training school. Now she works as our fistula advisor. She explains to patients who come in what a fistula is, or what an irreparable bladder is if they have that.

She's a new person. She changed 180 degrees. She's very religious, likes to dress up, and goes to church regularly. She also makes beautiful jewelry, which I take back to the US and try to sell for her. Unfortunately, a few years ago her sister died from hepatitis, and Memuna took in her two children. She's now raising them and paying for their schooling, and we pay for the place where they live.

Memuna has come into her own. It's so touching to see. Every day when I finish operating, she gets my scrub suit and washes and irons it. She is an inspiration to the staff and to the patients she works with.

https://youtu.be/DkDLSWhKFmE

• • •

Fina's story is similar to Memuna's. She was shunned from her village. People made fun of her, and she had to sleep in the barn with the goats and chickens.

She may be tiny, but Fina is a pistol. She also works for the West Africa Fistula Foundation, or WAFF. She eats at the hospital, and we pay for a place for her to stay. She, too, needed an opportunity to improve her life. She's a different person now.

https://youtu.be/dO2nOGt0Rxw

One lady went back to her village after we fixed her and said, "I'm dry." The villagers didn't believe her and went into her hut to check her bed. They couldn't believe it. She showed them that she was a new woman.

Can you imagine not ever being dry? Or not having running water? No towels? No electricity? Women with fistulas try to stay clean. They have to go to the river to wash their clothes and dry them in the sun, and as soon as they put them back on, they're wet again.

https://youtu.be/nFxDBs6ua9g

A few of the women who come to us thinking they have an obstetric fistula don't have one. What they have is a fistula of the bladder caused by cancer of the cervix, which eats a hole from the vagina to the bladder. There's nothing that can be done in a case like that, when there's advanced, terminal cancer.

I know a guy named Ishmael who comes by now and then and tries to sell me trinkets. One day he brought his niece to see me. She was a twenty-five-year-old girl, but she looked like she was forty. She had black plastic sacks wrapped with string all around her legs, her pelvis, and her abdomen to try to keep the urine and feces from getting all over. It took her ten minutes to take them all off. I examined her, and she had very advanced cervical cancer eating into her bladder and rectum.

It's been shown that 70% of invasive cervical cancer is caused by human papillomavirus, HPV, which is sexually transmitted. Certain strains are very aggressive. Sexual promiscuity in Africa is widespread, just as it is in the US. But at least in the US, we have screening mechanisms. In Sierra Leone, there are no pathologists. Even if a Pap smear was taken, there is no one in the country who could examine it under a microscope.

I met Mariama at the Princess Christian Maternity Hospital in Freetown. She knew she didn't have a fistula, but she knew she had a problem. As soon as I examined her, I knew she had very advanced cervical cancer. She was twenty-three at the time. When Mariama was sixteen, she had been captured by the rebels during the civil war and was raped, tortured, and dragged around the country. She managed to escape shortly before the war ended after three years in captivity.

I told Mariama that there was no surgical treatment for her. I called a cancer specialist, Dr. Larry Barker, and a radiation oncologist, Dr. Mary Hebert, whom I knew in the US, and they both said that if I brought Mariama to Texas, they would treat her for free.

I went to the US Embassy, where they knew me, and they gave me a visa for Mariama. But we couldn't get her an airline ticket on the same day as my flight. So she came by herself a week later, having never before been out of the country or on an airplane. Fortunately, she met a nice lady on the plane who helped her make the transfer in London. My wife and I picked Mariama up on a Saturday at Dallas/Fort Worth airport and took her home. She couldn't believe the house we lived in and wondered why there weren't fifteen or twenty people living there instead of just the three of us.

She was scheduled to see the doctors the second Monday after her arrival, in about nine days' time. The Sunday before her first appointment, at around 4:00 a.m., she came into our bedroom with blood pouring down her legs. She was in shock. I took her into the bathroom, put her in the bathtub, and had my wife hold her feet up in the air while I quickly got dressed. I put her over my shoulder, took her to the car, and drove her to the emergency room, which fortunately is only six blocks away from our house. Everyone in the emergency room knew me, even though I hadn't been practicing medicine there for six or seven years.

We started an IV, transfused her with four units of blood, and got the bleeding to stop. When the radiation oncologist saw Mariama on Monday, she said that we had to start radiation treatment immediately to shrink the tumor and prevent more bleeding. Chemotherapy was also started. After three months, in early December, I took Mariama home to Sierra Leone.

We knew that the radiation and chemotherapy probably didn't kill all of the tumor cells, but we were hoping for it. I did my surgeries, went back to Texas, and returned to Sierra Leone in late February. I examined Mariama again, and she had what we call persistence of disease, not a recurrence, because the cancer had never gone away. She was beginning to experience a lot of pain and wanted to go back to the US with me. She loved the luxury of having lights, running water, watching game shows on TV, being fed, and primarily, having pain relief.

We went to visit her family who lived in a small, shabby house. I talked to her mother, her boyfriend, and her brother, and they all agreed that Mariama should go back to the US with me. That was one of the saddest days of my life, seeing them say goodbye. They knew she wouldn't be coming back. They knew she was going to the US to die.

I got her a ticket and another visa. We landed at DFW airport and went through customs. Mariama couldn't speak English very well so I went up to the counter with her. Of course, she's black and I'm white. An African-American girl was the customs officer, and she demanded that I stand back behind the line. I yelled at her and said I was going to stay, so Mariama stepped back. I explained that Mariama had terminal cancer and that I was bringing her to the US to die. Then Mariama walked back to the counter and, in front of her, the customs officer said she'd let Mariama stay in the US for six months.

I said, "We need longer than six months."

And then the customs officer said, "Well, she's going

to die before six months, isn't she?"

I was livid. I couldn't believe she had said that in front of Mariama. I thought I was going to be thrown in jail, I was so mad. I reported the incident, but nothing ever came of it—very typical of our government.

Grayson County Home Hospice was there to provide the medication needed to make Mariama comfortable, and she was feeling good. My wife cooked for her every day. Mariama loved chicken, especially the bones. She would reach over to my plate, get the bones, and eat them, too. My wife did her laundry, made her bed, and cleaned up after her, even when the tumor was giving off a horrific odor. She did everything for her.

Mariama went to church with us every Sunday, sang solos, and got baptized. My wife took her shopping and bought her anything she wanted. Mariama couldn't believe the malls. She wore beautiful African dresses, which people loved, and went everywhere we went. Mariama touched so many people in our community.

Finally, about nine months later, in December, she started deteriorating. Hospice had been coming from the minute we had pulled up to the door of my house after returning from Africa, and now that she was having more pain, they checked on her every day. They were wonderful. They fell in love with Mariama, like everyone did. One nurse in particular, Anita Anderson, became very fond of her and gave her care beyond the call of duty. Amanda

Counce, a speech therapist, became so involved that she ended up going to Sierra Leone with me twice. To this day, she's supporting Mariama's stepdaughter. Tell me it is not a small world—I delivered Amanda's husband.

Finally, she needed twenty-four-hour care, and we put Mariama in a nursing home. She died on January 26. She was twenty-eight years old. She'd made it almost eleven months.

We buried Mariama in our family cemetery plot in Wilburton. The Stumpff family slipped around and paid the funeral expenses. There were probably 150 people at her funeral.

That's what medicine and life are all about—relationships and taking care of people.

Conclusion

"WHAT DO YOU HAVE TO GIVE?"

"Monkey see, monkey do."

I'd be lying if I said I didn't enjoy nice things. I make investments. I'm not going without food, shelter, or clothing because I'm giving everything away. But I am content. I have enough. I don't want any more.

My dad used to say that when you hear something enough times from older people, you better pay attention. Well, I heard "Basta! Basta!" Enough! What else do you need?

I learned by example. Both my father and my grandfather were very generous. I loved the phrase my dad used to say, "Monkey see, monkey do." I saw that my dad cared.

He buried Manuel Carter, the black man who lived in the shack, and paid for his funeral. He brought him food every Sunday. He never wanted anyone to know about it. It was just understood that that's what you're supposed to do. He used to thank God for hot water, which he didn't have as a kid. Nowadays we take things for granted. I keep lights on during the day because I love light. If my dad saw me doing that, he would have said that I was burning daylight.

There's a happy medium. There's a point when enough is enough. Before my father passed away, he was close to having renal failure and needed heart surgery. We drove out to the farm, and he looked across the land and said, "Son, I don't want to have heart surgery." He was seventy-eight years old at the time. "I've lived my life. I've always told you that you're not going to live forever on this earth." He looked down over the farm and the cattle and said, "I thank God for the opportunity to use this farm. It's not my farm. It's God's land. I thank God for the opportunity to have been able to use it." A year later, he died.

That's the legacy I got from my dad.

How are you going to give back? It doesn't have to be in Africa, but what are you going to do?

I'm not trying to tell people how to live, or what they should or shouldn't be doing. I'm far from perfect. I've made mistakes. Hopefully, I've learned from them, grown, and matured.

What anyone does to find gratification or happiness is an individual decision. Not everybody is supposed to go overseas to help people. You can do something meaningful in your community or in your church. My wife likes to take a fish dinner with coleslaw to the lady who lives by herself, several blocks from us. When she was delivering Meals on Wheels two or three times a week, she knew the names of all the pets and brought them treats. Once she found an old man without a working refrigerator and arranged for one to be delivered to his home. That's the way my wife gives. What's important is to find a way to help people.

We've got to give back. I found out that the more I give, the more I have.

Very few people in Sierra Leone knew about obstetric fistula when I started going there. Even the minister of health didn't know what it was. A lot of people today still don't know what it is, but more know now. The West Africa Fistula Foundation has definitely made an impact.

The key is prevention, because when you prevent a fistula, you're doing two things. One, you're saving a baby's life, and two, you're saving the mother's life by making sure she has access to a safe delivery. Timely intervention is essential. The most important thing is to educate people about what causes fistula and what can be done to avoid it. Today, after surgery, many women are able to go back to their villages. More and more families are willing to take them back. Husbands and villagers are learning about what caused the fistula, and that it isn't a curse, as many people still believe.

Education, economics, jobs, and spreading the word are all key. My goal is to create sustainability.

When I first went to Sierra Leone, seven or eight students a year were graduating from medical school due to the war that had just ended. Today, about thirty-five students graduate annually, but 95% of them leave the country. They go somewhere else to work because there are no facilities, they get paid hardly anything, and there's no one to give them specialized training. There is a phenomenal need for all these things.

• • •

Ever since I started working in Bo, I have had the dream to create a medical center, a true medical center on par with the Mayo Clinic or Cleveland Clinic. I call it the West Africa Medical Center. It could be a charity hospital, just like the one in New Orleans. I already have a logo, a website, and land.

A young man whom we had hired to help redo one of the wards told me about Bandajuma, his wife's village, which is along the highway about seven kilometers east of Bo. Over a period of a few years, from about 2009 to 2012, we acquired sixty-five acres of land in Bandajuma. We didn't pay an outrageous price, but we built a schoolhouse in the village that cost us over $17,000. About 400 students go there now. During the Ebola crisis, we sent the villagers money to pay for food and bleach so they wouldn't have to leave their village. Fortunately, no one died in Bandajuma. In a village three kilometers away, thirty-five people were lost to Ebola.

I want to build a center for training medical students and young doctors on how to do C-sections, hysterectomies, and to care for obstetric patients so doctors will stay in Sierra Leone. I want them to have training, too, in general surgery, orthopedic surgery, neurosurgery, plastic surgery, heart surgery, cardiology, nephrology, internal medicine—everything. All those doctors in the US who get fed up with medicine and retire early like me could come to teach. Then they'd get their calling back and feel gratification.

I want to help through education. I want to help people jump start their lives, not be just a for-free charity. Training doctors will help Sierra Leoneans help themselves and stimulate the economy. I think everyone wants to get out of bed, go to work, and be a productive citizen. I'd rather teach someone to fish rather than give them a fish. If I create dependency, then I have failed them.

I want to build the West Africa Medical Center one step at a time and then, in ten or fifteen or twenty years, I'll turn it over to Sierra Leoneans and leave. They'll be the experts then. I want people from all over West Africa to refer patients to the Center. I want to include a cancer center, cardiology, and kidney dialysis, but very first of all, the specialties will be obstetrics, because so many women are dying needlessly every day.

We could have people from Australia, Canada, England, or Germany come to the Center and pay to do research and development. Why go to London or Liverpool to study tropical medicine? The tropical diseases are there, in Sierra Leone: schistosomiasis, malaria, Lassa fever, Ebola, leishmaniasis, and leprosy.

That's my vision. There is so much good we could do.

The West Africa Fistula Foundation is not just me. It's always been a team: the people who scrub the floors, the people who cook the meals, the nurses, people who clean the instruments; the guys who drive the vehicles out to get the patients, and Paul, who helped build the hospital and keeps the generator running so we have light for doing surgeries. It's a whole team.

We have a gentleman working with us who has a tremendous passion to help people. His name is Peacemaker, and he's based in Kabala, in the northern part of Sierra Leone. He's not a nurse but has always been very active in health care. We send him out to the villages on what we call sensitization trips. We bought him a motorcycle so the he can go way back into the bush. He even goes into Guinea.

Peacemaker doesn't work exclusively for WAFF. He's also extremely active at the clinic in Kabala, where they do deliveries and treat all kinds of illnesses. The staff at the clinic are smart enough to realize that if ladies can't deliver to send them to the hospital right away for a C-section. Peacemaker also finds fistula patients for us. At one point, he had as many as fifteen patients living in his house until he could manage to bring them to Bo. He's truly dedicated, highly motivated, and a wonderful guy.

In *The Different Drum*, Scott Peck writes that the first thing to do when you obtain power is to disperse it. It's human nature to abuse power, he says. And that's so true. I've been told that I'm a good leader. That's because I give people responsibility. I let them shine. It's always a team approach.

One of the most important things I've learned in my life is that we're all the same. When I cut through skin doing surgery, whether it's black, white, brown, or yellow, there's no difference inside. The only difference between the people in Sierra Leone and those of us born in the US is that they were born there. We all have the same needs and the same basic wants.

Most people in Sierra Leone are content and happy with what they have even though, in my opinion, they have so little. They don't know anything else. They don't know about running water, electricity, being able to take a shower inside the house, having adequate food, or eating meals at a table with chairs. Many Sierra Leoneans sleep on the ground. They don't know any different, but that doesn't mean I don't want to try to improve their lives, improve their longevity, and give them an opportunity to help themselves. They're so appreciative of anything we do for them. For example, when we buy a patient a Coke, she won't open it. She'll put it on the nightstand and take it back to her village to show everyone.

There are a tremendous number of people, in all races, who are decent, and there are also a lot of people in all races who are evil. Hopefully, before I leave this earth, there will be more decent people than those who aren't.

When I go to Africa, Jim Stewart, an old friend who grew up three doors down from me, makes sure I buy ice cream for the kids. He gives me money every trip just for ice cream for kids in the neighborhood. They've never seen ice cream in their life, and they love it. Something so simple means so much to them. And to see the toys they play with! They take a gas can, cut it in two, use lids for wheels, and make themselves a little car. They are so happy. Another thing they love playing with is a worn-out bicycle tire and a stick. They roll it around all day long. These kids are happy with such simple things.

When I go out to eat and spend $25 on a meal for my wife and granddaughter, I think to myself, "My God, what I could do with $25 in Sierra Leone."

If I could wake people up in the United States to realize when enough is enough—basta!—there's so much more that we could do.

I feel very blessed to have had the upbringing I did. I give all the credit to my father and grandfather. If they hadn't provided me with a solid foundation, I wouldn't have been able to achieve the things I have in my life. Now it's up to me to continue their legacy and to help my fellow human beings.

The only way to find happiness, pleasure, or gratification is by giving, not giving to get but giving unselfishly. To be able to say, "Basta! I have enough! Now I want to give."

There are so many people in this world who are suffering, and there are so many ways all of us can give.

The only time I'll be done is when I never again see another fistula in Sierra Leone.

Basta for now!

Deno's Wisdom

SAYINGS FROM MY FATHER

- When you're healthy, you're wealthy.
- Always have an understanding to avoid a misunderstanding.
- You have another think coming.
- Don't let someone put their head on your shoulder.
- It's easy to spend someone else's money.
- The less you say, the less you have to take back.
- It's easy to buy something but hard to pay for it.
- Death is a great equalizer.
- Can't get something for nothing.
- Memory is so short. (Pertaining primarily to how we almost lost our freedom during WW II)
- Easy come, easy go.

- You must start somewhere and if it's at the top, there's only one way to go: down!
- A penny saved is a penny earned.
- There are always consequences to our actions, good or bad.
- If you run around with a bunch of jackasses, you'll never make it to the Kentucky Derby.
- Paddle your own canoe.
- Right will always win out!

Acknowledgments

I feel guilty sometimes, but not for long, because practicing medicine was fulfilling. The number of friends I have been so fortunate to develop over the years is no doubt in the tens of thousands. There is not one day I do not think of or see one of my former patients, their husbands, or the children I delivered, and it is so neat to visit with them or one of their relatives. Of course I will never forget the ones who have passed away or had significant health issues (mental and physical), which opens up those very sad and depressive wounds we experienced together.

I just want to thank you for allowing me to be part of your life and hope I contributed to your life in a positive way.

My office staff was so loyal and dedicated to the ultimate goal, and that was "taking care of the patient." They always answered the phone (and not make you talk to an answering machine, heaven forbid), stayed late until the last patient was seen, returned every phone call from that day, and called as soon as we got a patient's lab test, mammogram or pap smear back. We were a team. We all laughed together and of course cried together when things did not go as planned.

Numerous nurses, aides, cleaners, maintenance men, and other hospital personnel put up with my idiosyncrasies, but we sure had some wonderful times laughing when at 2: 00 a.m. I came up out of the linen cart and scared Legacy while she was mopping, or tried to run over Roger in the postal jeep I used to drive, or crawled on the floor under the bed of a post-op patient in the recovery room we had just operated on in the middle of the night and grabbed Peggy's leg, which made her scream and run down the hall.

Peggy Kean comes to mind because for twenty-plus years I have wanted to write this book but obviously the timing was not there and we did not force it. Peggy transcribed from my dictation over 400 pages of single-spaced ideas and thoughts I had expressed over the years, many at 2:00 a.m. while I was waiting for a lady to deliver and many when I would wake at 3:00 a.m. and think "I must write this down."

The African experience has opened up a new chapter in my life and I could go on and on, but know if I tried I'm going to miss mentioning someone. The Board of West

Africa Fistula Foundation, Shawn Graft who accompanied his wife Dr. Alex Rogers to Sierra Leone and now for years has volunteered to use his technology skills with the website and to straighten out regular newsletters sent via email. Kurt Stumpff and family have been so instrumental in their encouragement and financial support. Dr. Susan Hardwick-Smith, an extremely busy OB-GYN with a huge practice in Houston and a fireball of a person with phenomenal energy and support. She also has been to Sierra Leone several times.

A special thanks to Dr. Neil Shulman who has encouraged and prodded me to write this book ASAP.

Numerous volunteers include Helen Weld, a very dedicated and loyal nurse who helped for years and left a trail of tears every time she went for home to get some rest. Julia Robinson a very hard working young lady who manned the ship for several months. Isaac Van Bebber (I remember when she was in her mother's car seat when her older brother came to play with my son) at a young age came to Sierra Leone and ruled with a commander's spirit. Now she is a naval officer aboard a ship, carrying on her goal of protecting our country. Jennifer Bennett from Australia, an amazing, very positive and talented lady with a background of surgical nurse, midwife, and administrator. Kathi Beasley, a videographer and writer who accompanied Dr. Susan Hardwick-Smith and spent countless hours putting together video and pictures so we could show the rest of the world what it is really like in Sierra Leone.

We have had numerous college students, some now in medical school, others who have become doctors, nurses, and obviously numerous practicing doctors who have come to help out. Dr. Rex Hubbard, whom I met at Texoma Medical Center when I took Mariama to the hospital when she was in shock and bleeding so badly. He was doing locum work and decided to come to Sierra Leone and hopefully will be back soon with his twin brother who is an anesthesiologist. Dr. Robert Kester has been to Sierra Leone several times and has been very supportive and involved in producing and paying for our calendars. Dr. Clifford Wheeless, a world-renowned gynecological oncologist and author of many textbooks who helped initially with the urinary diversions. Dr. Jay Smith, a world-renowned urological oncologist who helped with the urinary diversions and is chairman of the Department of Urology at Vanderbilt Medical Center. Dr. Mark and Margaret Hyslop from Canada, whom I met in Sierra Leone in 2010 and who have been so supportive of and active in our organization. Dr. Mark taught at Njalla University in Bo a few years ago.

So many donors, even many from Europe, who heard of us and sent donations ranging from $2 to $10,000 and had faith that we would be good stewards of their monies. Other donors: Leila Janah and Shirvani Garg with Samahope, Betty Seaborn with daughters Linda Templin and Jennifer Seaborn of the Idea Foundation, Amanda Paniaqua and Nell with Medshare, and John Lyon and Carrie Jo Cain of World Hope. Patty Hoskin from England, a nurse who has gone several times to help and even with her husband's health gives talks and holds luncheons to raise money and send to our organization on a regular basis. Carolyn Emery, a longtime school mate who is extremely talented in writing and wonders what happened to me as we had the same English teacher Mrs. Odis Quaid.

I could not go without mentioning Jimi Lou Coleman, my office manager and the one who quotes scripture to me when things seem insurmountable.

I also send my thanks to the team at Book In A Box, for helping make this book a reality.

Last but not least, my sincere appreciation for all of the phenomenal talent and hard work that Andrea and Paul Robinson have put in to help West Africa Fistula Foundation and the people of Sierra Leone. All of this reaffirms there are some great people and that it does take a team. There is no I in TEAM!

I know I forgot someone but please forgive me.

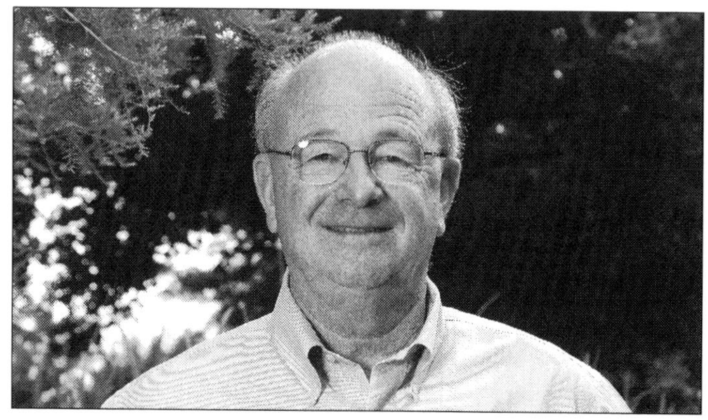

About the Author

After a successful twenty-two-year career as an OB-GYN, Dr. Darius Maggi founded the West Africa Fistula Foundation in 2004. He currently spends much of his time and mission with a focus on Sierra Leone, where he brings help to women who don't otherwise have access to safe, modern health care. Dr. Maggi credits his Italian immigrant grandfather and his blue-collar father as the source of his selfless dedication in the service of others. One hundred percent of the proceeds of *Basta!* go toward support of the Foundation's goal to establish proper treatment and care for this devastating condition.

The author of this book writes about the values and ethics he learned as a child and how these two were incorporated into his daily life with virtually everyone he met. I had the privilege of working with Dr. Maggi for approximately 22 years, and witnessed daily his love and genuine concern for his patients. His work ethic was like no other, he would stay after office hours to see sick patients, even those who had no means to pay, or those who would barter for care, with either a package of fish or fresh vegetables. His patients always seemed better after seeing him, sometimes, just by his humor alone. I'll never forget the day he came in and announced, "Basta! Basta!" I was shocked, but also felt fortunate to have had his daily encouragement throughout the years. In fact, that is why I chose to become a Registered Nurse. After attaining my RN degree, I worked alongside him, in the hospital setting, helping to bring thousands of babies into this world. All of his patients absolutely loved him. To this day, I still hear praise from his prior patients, as they await the birth of their grandchildren. I have remained personable and focused on patient care, but with technology continually taking over the medical field, it is getting more and more difficult to do. I am still saddened by Dr. Maggi saying "BASTA! BASTA!" but completely understand. Dr. Maggi continues to show his love for human life by helping women in Africa. These women are truly blessed to be in his God gifted hands.

— KATHY CROWLEY, RNC, LABOR AND DELIVERY

Compassionate, kind, respectful, giving, personable, motivational, workaholic, and humorous, the list could go on forever; however, these are just a few of many words I think of, to describe Dr. Maggi. I had the privilege of working with him approximately 20 years and remember so clearly the day he said, "Basta, Basta!" I was overcome with sadness and grief, almost as if there had been a death in the family. I knew I would never again work with a person such as him. His true love and respect for humankind was like no other. His actions spoke louder than words and he lived by the principle of treating others like you want to be treated. His presence would simply light up the room and paired with his humor, he would put a smile on everyone's face. In fact, I smile now as I reminisce on his uniqueness. I feel honored to have known and worked with Dr. Maggi—he was one of a kind.

— KATHY WILLIAMS, RNC, LABOR AND DELIVERY

Darius Maggi, MD deftly wields a sharp scalpel to accomplish his surgical cures in Sierra Leone, West Africa yet his homespun wisdom and captivating experiences may initiate the more complex cure for today's doubters and despondent people. So if you are seeking a sermon, don't bother. But if an inspirational message is on your menu, then pull up a chair and read awhile. Basta!

— TIM BRUMIT, MD, FAAP, FRIEND AND COLLEAGUE OF THIRTY-FOUR YEARS

Made in the USA
Columbia, SC
26 March 2018